VEGAN KETO

60+ High-Fat Plant-Based Recipes to Nourish Your Mind & Body

Liz MacDowell

VICTORY BELT PUBLISHING
Las Vegas

First Published in 2018 by Victory Belt Publishing Inc.

ISBN-13: 978-1-628603-14-9

The author is not a licensed practitioner, physician, or medical professional and offers no medical diagnoses, treatments, suggestions, or counseling. The information presented herein has not been evaluated by the U.S. Food and Drug Administration, and it is not intended to diagnose, treat, cure, or prevent any disease. Full medical clearance from a licensed physician should be obtained before beginning or modifying any diet, exercise, or lifestyle program, and physicians should be informed of all nutritional changes.

The author/owner claims no responsibility to any person or entity for any liability, loss, or damage caused or alleged to be caused directly or indirectly as a result of the use, application, or interpretation of the information presented herein.

Front and back cover photos by Hayley Mason and Bill Staley

Cover design by Justin-Aaron Velasco

Interior design by Yordan Terziev and Boryana Yordanova

Printed in Canada

TC 0623

Contents

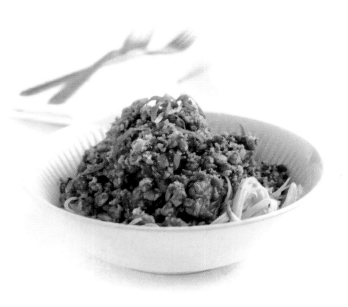

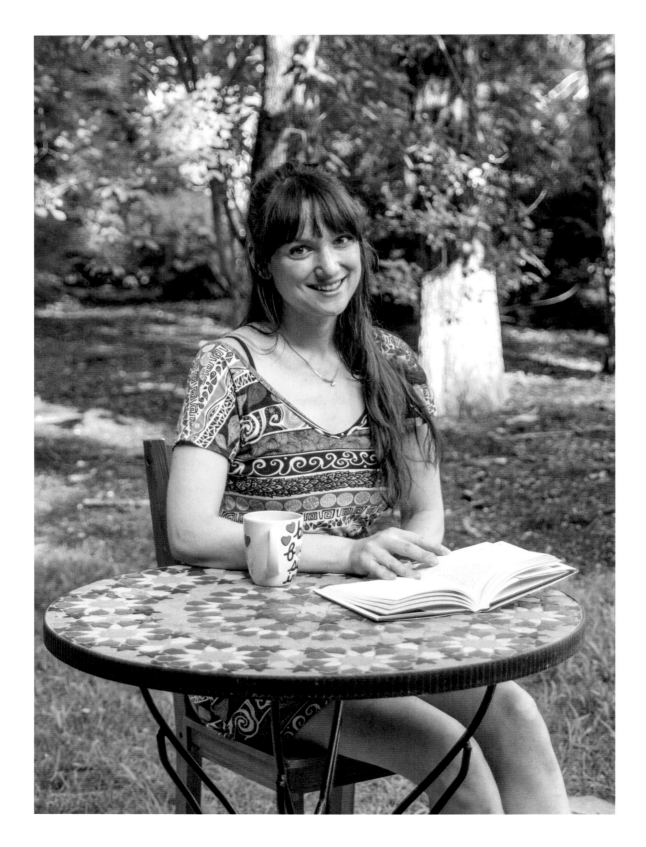

About This Book

As ketogenic diets grow in popularity, it is becoming increasingly apparent that there is no single "right" way to achieve and maintain ketosis. Many popular voices in the keto space offer a perspective that differs from the traditional, more dogmatic approach to low-carb eating. It has been really cool to watch the popularity of this diet grow over the years and to see the different strategies, tips, and even products that members of the keto community dream up.

When I first started keto as a vegan, there weren't many resources out there for those of us who don't eat meat (or eggs or dairy), so I started blogging at *Meat Free Keto* as a way to share my experiences and the silly recipes I came up with. I thought that maybe the information could help a few other people out there get started eating in this way that has been so transformative for me.

Over the years, the way I choose to practice keto and low-carb eating has certainly evolved. As I dove deeper into learning about nutrition, I began to adapt my keto diet strategy to focus more on nutrient density and ingredient quality. It's almost embarrassing to look back on how I ate in the beginning, but everyone has to start somewhere, right?

I've made plenty of mistakes over the past six years, and I've also discovered lots of little tricks to make keto easier. The information in this book is the culmination of all that gained knowledge, insight, and experience. I hope that this book can make your transition to a plant-based keto diet as easy as possible while providing some tasty recipes along the way.

Why I Tried Keto

There's a common saying that it takes 10,000 hours to master a skill. Assuming this is true, I am most definitely a master of dieting. For the better part of two decades, I've spent a pretty embarrassing amount of time worrying about my weight, my pants size, the amount of food I ate, the amount of food I didn't eat, and how many calories I could burn in a given day.

As you can probably guess, I've tried a few different diets. In addition to the mainstream programs that have you count points or purchase branded meals and shakes, I've dipped my toes in somewhat more extreme dieting waters. I've tried high-carb raw vegan diets, with 80 percent of calories coming from fruits and vegetables. I've tried juice fasts, where all you consume for weeks at a time is fresh-pressed juice. And I've tried extreme calorie restriction, limiting my intake to just 500 calories per day—while running 5 to 10 miles daily to try to keep my weight within the "normal" range.

None of these approaches proved to be particularly successful or sustainable. Sure, I lost weight with each trendy new diet (with the exception of the high-carb raw vegan diet), but I felt awful, and I always gained everything back once I could no longer keep up the momentum.

Each of those diets felt like a fight with my body. I spent the majority of my time thinking about all the food I wasn't eating, focusing on the gnawing hunger in my gut, and chugging diet soda and black coffee to try to make it through the day on what little nutrition I was willing to allow myself. I wasted so much brainpower trying to calculate calories consumed versus calories burned, the timing of meals for the most effective fat burning, the overall "goodness" and "badness" of various foods based on whichever arbitrary statistic seemed important at the moment, and how

fast/far/long I would have to run in order to "afford" whatever it was that I'd just eaten.

Let me tell you, it was *exhausting*.

This was my approach to diet and nutrition for more than ten years, and it definitely didn't do me any favors. My digestion, which had been pretty rocky my entire life, continued to worsen into my twenties, and I seemed to catch every bug that went around. I was tired, hungry, and sick of feeling awful all the time, both physically and emotionally.

I wanted to escape the cycle of dieting, but I honestly had no idea how to do it. I felt trapped—as soon as I stopped restricting, I would gain weight, but constantly depriving myself wasn't proving to be an overwhelmingly successful plan, either.

In the spring of 2012, I found high-carb raw veganism and ran with it. It seemed like the answer to all my problems. Proponents of this way of eating suggested that you didn't have to track calories or worry about the nutritional content of what you were eating. As long as you ate to satiation, your body would get the appropriate nutrition and you would be at your set weight. But this wasn't the case for me. At all.

I gained weight pretty much immediately, despite eating just fruit, lots of greens, and some nuts. I was hungry, irritable, and cold all the time... in the middle of July. I felt exhausted and sick, too, but I kept going because every "guru" I encountered and read about online insisted that this was the perfect human diet, and soon I would start to feel amazing. I stuck it out for a little over a month before I threw in the towel and started to look for a better way.

Like so many others, I found out about ketogenic diets via the internet. In fact, I found out about keto while browsing weight loss progress pictures on Reddit one night. Having just stopped eating a high-carb raw vegan diet due because of how terrible it made me feel, my interest in a better way to diet was definitely piqued.

I saw so many dramatic before-and-after photos, all touting keto as the secret to those results. After spending the night poring over the keto subreddit, I decided to give it a shot. After all, I had just discovered that high-carb wasn't the way to go for me. Why not try the opposite approach?

I went all-in.

I noticed results pretty quickly. I dropped 5 pounds in the first week. After three months, I had lost the 20 pounds that were plaguing me, all without making any other changes to my lifestyle.

Aside from the weight loss, I noticed other improvements in my well-being. My digestion had normalized for the first time in my life. While going gluten-free earlier in the year had certainly helped ease my symptoms of irritable bowel syndrome (IBS), keto brought about a dramatic change in how my digestive system functioned. Without going into too many details, let me just say that I finally understood what doctors and fiber supplement ads mean when they talk about being "regular."

In addition to the digestive changes, I experienced a decrease in joint pain and swelling—symptoms I didn't even realize I had until they weren't there anymore. I woke up feeling well rested, found that I could think more clearly, and even had more energy throughout the day.

Not all the changes occurred so quickly.

After several months of eating a ketogenic diet, I started to notice my symptoms of endometriosis becoming less severe. For those who are unfamiliar with endometriosis, it's a menstrual disorder that causes a lot of pain and swelling and mood imbalances (among a host of other issues). While the pain and swelling haven't disappeared entirely, these symptoms are usually mild enough that I can live normally instead of being unable to get out of bed several days each month.

By contrast, I also started noticing how terrible eating excessive carbs made my body feel. Like so many others, my first shot at keto was not the only one. I would grow bored, or lazy, or I would say "just this once" about a certain food and then find myself continuing to indulge in high-carb treats for the next week. Each time this happened, I'd feel awful and hungover for days from the sugar and high carb intake and would find myself crawling back toward low-carb eating.

Eventually, I realized that for me, keto isn't so much a diet as a lifestyle, and I started treating it accordingly. Instead of trying to sneak in sugary foods and cheat the system, I began creating more "fun" recipes so that I wouldn't become bored or feel like I was missing out on desserts or little treats. I started looking at foods differently, focusing on how they made me feel rather than how they tasted. I stopped beating myself up over exceeding my carb limit on some days and shifted my attention to my overall eating habits and making positive choices on a larger scale. This strategy really helps me stay motivated to eat low-carb almost all the time, which makes me feel healthier and happier.

While I was learning all about keto from the internet, I was also enrolled in a nutrition program. Over time, I worked to combine this newfound nutrition knowledge with both my vegan diet and the ketogenic diet and started dialing in an approach that is effective and sustainable for me.

What Is a Ketogenic Diet?

In a nutshell, a ketogenic diet is a high-fat, low-carbohydrate, moderate-protein way of eating that shifts your body from burning glucose (sugar) for energy to a state of ketosis, in which your body preferentially uses ketone bodies and fat as a fuel source. Your liver creates ketone bodies from fat when your body needs to make energy but no glucose is present. This process most commonly occurs during periods of carbohydrate restriction, very limited food intake, and intense exercise. Acetoacetate and beta-hydroxybutyrate are ketone bodies; acetone (a by-product of their breakdown) is often considered a ketone body as well.

Most people in the world right now are burning glucose as their primary source of energy. When you eat something with carbohydrates in it, your body breaks down those carbs into simple sugars, the majority of which is glucose. This glucose is absorbed into your bloodstream, where it triggers the release of insulin by your pancreas. Insulin then calls for the uptake of glucose by your muscles to store that glucose for use as glycogen. Insulin also signals your body to store excess glucose and triglycerides as body fat and halts any fat burning currently going on.[1]

Fructose, the sugar commonly found in fruits, agave nectar, and—somewhat infamously—high-fructose corn syrup (among other foods), is processed by the liver, where it is either converted to glucose and sent to the bloodstream (where the above process takes place) or stored as fat (triglycerides)[2] in the liver. Though a very small amount of fructose is converted to triglycerides, over time, consuming extremely excessive amounts of fructose can lead to non-alcoholic fatty liver disease.[3]

While some people can go their entire lives burning glucose for fuel without issue, others have problems relying on glucose for energy. For starters, because the body can store only so much glycogen, you need to replenish those stores by eating often. You know that hangry feeling you get sometimes (read: all the time)? That's a by-product of your blood sugar crashing in the absence of sugar.[4] Mood swings and mood disorders are a surprisingly common side effect of blood sugar dysregulation,[5] and if you are anything like me, you are already well aware of this fact (as is any person who has ever lived with you).

If you've heard of insulin resistance, then you are already aware of another potential issue with burning glucose as your primary source of energy. Over time, overconsumption of carbohydrates can cause your tissues to become less sensitive to the insulin that your pancreas releases. Because the same amount of insulin is no longer achieving the desired effect, your poor pancreas starts to produce *more* insulin, which just perpetuates this cycle.

In the presence of insulin resistance, circulating glucose levels can remain too high, damaging tissues, keeping the body in a state of fat storage, and preventing the body from burning fat that has already been stored. Eventually, insulin resistance can lead to type 2 diabetes, other metabolic issues, and even cardiovascular disease.[6]

On the flip side of this equation, when there is too *little* circulating glucose in your bloodstream, the release of another hormone called glucagon is triggered. Glucagon tells your liver to convert that stored glycogen back to glucose for use as fuel. Glucagon also tells your body to break down stored fat into free fatty acids for use as fuel. Burning free fatty acids produces ketone bodies, which your brain and body can then use for energy. This is the beginning of nutritional ketosis. If you continue to restrict carbohydrates, your body will continue burning fat as its main fuel source.

Now, something cool about ketone metabolism is that it cuts insulin out of the picture. Instead of fluctuating, insulin and blood sugar levels remain relatively stable. This stability curbs fat storage, reduces food cravings, and promotes the breakdown of body fat.[7]

This ease of fat loss and regulation of hunger signals is one of the main reasons so many people (myself included) find themselves sticking with ketogenic and low-carb diets.

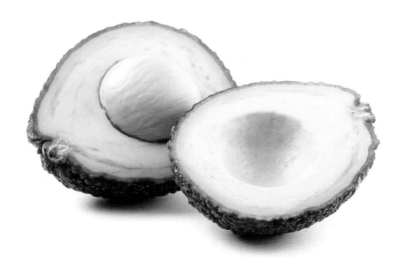

What Keto Isn't

There are a lot of misconceptions about ketogenic diets floating around, so I wanted to take a moment to address a few of the most common ones.

Ketosis Is Not Ketoacidosis

I think this is the biggest misconception I see perpetuated on the internet (and by some reputable-sounding sources, too!). Ketosis is a natural process that the body enters in response to carbohydrate restriction. It is thought to be an evolutionary development to provide protection from the effects of famine or food shortages.

Ketoacidosis is a very serious condition brought on by extremely high blood glucose levels combined with a severe lack of insulin. This rare condition can occur in type 1 diabetics but is very unlikely to occur in those without diabetes.[8]

Keto Is Not a Meat-Heavy Diet

I receive a lot of emails and social media comments expressing confusion that my diet is both vegan and ketogenic, as if the two were mutually exclusive. Because most portrayals of keto approach it from the "burgers, bacon, and cheese" side, there is a bit of uncertainty about the types of food you can eat.

As you probably figured (since this book is called *Vegan Keto*), you don't *have* to eat meat. You don't have to eat eggs, or dairy, or anything else you don't want to, either. A ketogenic diet is just a way of eating that gets you into ketosis; which types of foods you use to do so are totally up to you.

Keto Is Not a No-Carb Diet

There are "zero-carb diets" out there, where people mostly just eat meat. Some choose to add eggs or oil, but overall, the goal is to consume zero carbohydrates.

While this is a form of a ketogenic diet, it is by no means representative of all ketogenic diets. No-carb diets are on the extreme end of the spectrum. Most people following a ketogenic diet consume between 20 and 50 grams of net carbohydrates per day. (See pages 26 to 28 for more on net carbs.) When you factor in fiber, you could be eating as much as 100 grams of total carbohydrates!

I think this is an important distinction to make because I have seen many people argue against ketogenic diets, citing how they are too extreme in their total elimination of carbohydrates. For most people, this is simply not true.

Keto Is Not "One Size Fits All"

There is no one right way to do a ketogenic diet. Our bodies, lifestyles, and goals are all different, and so are the ways we approach eating. Some people choose to consume specific ratios of fat, protein, and carbohydrate, while others choose to count carbs. Some people prefer to take a more intuitive approach to keto and stick to eating foods that are lower in carbs and make them feel good.

As long as you are eating a diet that keeps you in a state of ketosis, you are eating keto. To find out how to tell if you are in ketosis, read the section about testing for ketones on pages 37 and 38.

Keto Is Not a List of Foods

 I can't stress this enough—ketogenic diets are not a list of foods you "can" or "cannot" have. I don't think it's helpful long-term to attach "goodness" or some sort of dietary morality to any certain food or set of foods. Instead, I think it's more valuable to assess foods on an individual basis and to evaluate what they do for (or to) our bodies. So, instead of saying, "You can't eat candy on keto," look at candy for what it is—mostly sugar, along with some industrial fats—and think about the impact eating it will have.

Saying you can't have a food because it's "not keto" turns the ketogenic diet into some sort of hyper-restrictive, dogmatic fad that places the onus on willpower for success. This model hasn't worked for most of us in the past, so why would it work now?

Of course, in the beginning, some people find it very helpful to keep a list of keto-friendly foods around until they are accustomed to the ketogenic way of eating (which is why there's a shopping list on pages 48 and 49 of this book!). There's nothing wrong with using a list if that's what works for you. Just be aware that there is no hard-and-fast list of "keto foods" out there.

Keto Is Not a High-Protein Diet

 The low-carb diets that have been popular in the past have also featured high amounts of protein. Ketogenic diets are different in that they do not prioritize consuming a lot of protein, because excess protein can be converted to glucose in the body (via a process called gluconeogenesis) and can kick you out of ketosis, mitigating the positive effects of the diet.[9]

Keto Is Not a Silver Bullet

I think it's important to set reasonable expectations. It's easy to get caught up in the excitement of seeing striking weight loss results in online forums and hearing people's stories of turning their lives and health around. For some, a keto diet can be life-changing, but not everyone has such a dramatic experience.

We all want that quick-and-easy answer, and while some people do experience drastic changes quite quickly, that's not the case for everyone. So don't get frustrated if you don't see results instantly!

Is Butter a Carb?
Taking a Look at Macronutrients

It's hard to talk about ratios of macronutrients without first identifying what macronutrients are. Macronutrients, or "macros" for short, are the three main components that make up all foods—fat, protein, and carbohydrate. Our bodies use these macronutrients for energy, breaking them down into usable parts and storing the excess as body fat for periods of scarcity. These three subjects are pretty complex and involve a lot of moving parts, but I'm just going to cover the basics for now.

Carbs Are Not Actually the Devil

It's easy to get carried away and classify all carbohydrates as bad, but that's oversimplifying things a bit. Carbohydrates (and even sugars) are natural components in plants, and therefore in the foods we eat. The key is not to avoid carbohydrates altogether, but to choose the carbohydrates that give you the most nutritional bang for your buck.

In a standard Western diet, most of the carbohydrates come from processed grains or starches and refined sugars. In a vegan ketogenic way of eating, the majority of carbohydrates come from nuts, seeds, greens, nonstarchy vegetables, and some berries.

Once I became fat-adapted, I stopped worrying about the carbohydrates I eat in the form of dark leafy greens and crunchy veggies like broccoli, cauliflower, celery, cucumbers, and radishes. Yes, those foods are carbohydrates, but I find that the nutritional benefits of having an extra serving of broccoli at dinner outweigh the downsides of getting a few extra grams of net carbs.

Fruit is another topic that stirs up loud opinions in the keto sphere. In short, yes, you can eat fruit. Most fruits are pretty high in carbs, but berries are relatively low and contain antioxidants, as well as vitamins and minerals. So, if you're going to enjoy fruit on keto, berries are a good choice.

Some people avoid fruit while they are becoming fat-adapted. Doing so isn't necessary as long as you are eating few enough carbohydrates to stay in ketosis, but it can make maintaining ketosis a bit easier. You can also choose to minimize carb consumption and avoid fruits and most vegetables in the early stage. It's really up to you.

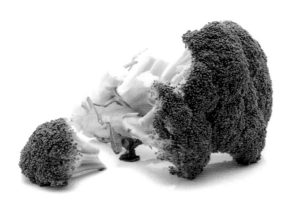

BUT . . . YOU *NEED* CARBS!

A lot of nutrition professionals (and people with expensive-enough recording equipment to seem like professionals on YouTube) claim that you need carbs to live. Your brain functions on them! You will die without carbs!

This isn't necessarily untrue, but it's pretty misleading. The simple truth is that there are no essential carbohydrates, like there are essential amino acids and essential fatty acids that you need to eat in order to function. Your brain does need some carbohydrates, but it doesn't need you to eat carbs to get them.

Remember that bit about your body turning excess protein (amino acids) into glucose via gluconeogenesis? Well, this mechanism exists for a reason. Should your body require more glucose than you are eating in the form of carbohydrates, it is perfectly capable of creating its own supply.

A Quick Intro to Fats

The topic of fats is not just complicated; it's incredibly controversial and heavily debated in the public sphere on a daily basis. Much of the negative press about the ketogenic diet, for instance, centers around shock at the sheer quantity of fat that keto dieters consume. After all, we were raised to think that dietary fat is the cause of so many health issues, from obesity to cardiovascular disease.

When I first read about the seemingly insane amount of fat that those on a ketogenic diet regularly eat, I was similarly perplexed. I had spent most of my life focusing on eating low-fat and fat-free foods, trying to fit into the smallest size possible, and now I was reading that a high-fat diet might actually be the answer. I felt a mix of equal parts annoyance and curiosity.

As I learned more about dietary fat, I realized that it was ridiculous to have avoided it for so long. Fats, and especially the whole foods that contain them, are loaded with vitamins, minerals, and other phytochemicals that are essential to our health. Additionally, studies show that diets like the Mediterranean diet that are higher in fats (particularly those in olives and olive oil, but also those from fish and some cheeses) can be protective of both heart and brain health.[10]

Sources of Fat

Years ago, I worked as a "healthy eating specialist" at a natural grocery chain. The job involved making healthy recipes and educating both employees and customers on the benefits of various foods. While the program on the whole was a bit fat-phobic, one part of the philosophy stuck with me—to prioritize obtaining fats from whole-food sources.

The idea behind this recommendation is that an olive provides more nutrition than olive oil and that tahini (a paste made of ground sesame seeds) brings more to the table than sesame oil. I took this information to heart and have incorporated it into the way I eat and cook. That's not to say I don't use oils at all; I just try to think about whether I could incorporate the whole food into the meal instead.

Plant sources of fat on a ketogenic diet include avocados, coconut, olives, nuts, seeds, and their oils. For a more complete list, take a look at page 48.

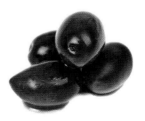

Saturated Fats Versus MUFAs Versus PUFAs

There are a lot of acronyms when it comes to fats, and it can get a little confusing. To simplify the issue, let's take a quick look at the different types of fats and their sources:

- **Saturated fatty acids (SFAs)** are solid at room temperature. They tend to oxidize slowly because of their structure.† Vegans typically find saturated fats in coconut (along with coconut oil), palm oil, and cocoa butter.

- **Monounsaturated fats (MUFAs)** are generally liquid at room temperature but become solid in the fridge. Avocados, nuts, olives, and the oils from these foods are sources of MUFAs. These oils are the ones typically used for cooking.

- **Polyunsaturated fats (PUFAs)** remain liquid even when refrigerated and are far more delicate than MUFAs or saturated fats. Therefore, they should not be used for cooking and are better obtained from whole-food sources. Essential fatty acids (like omega-3s and omega-6s) are PUFAs. Sources of PUFAs include the oils derived from flax and most seeds and industrial oils, like canola (rapeseed) oil, corn oil, and other "vegetable oils" (see the sidebar below).

Buying & Storing Oils

I try to buy extra-virgin, cold-pressed oils (which come from the first pressing) whenever possible, as these oils have a higher nutrient content than the oils from the second or third pressing, as well as those that have been processed with high heat.

Regardless of the type, I like to store oils in a cool, dark place. I store seeds and oils that are high in PUFAs in the fridge and avoid large temperature shifts to prevent oxidation.

Cooking with Oils

For cooking, I prioritize using either coconut oil or olive oil. You can certainly use other MUFAs for cooking, but I find them to be cost-prohibitive. I also try to keep the heat on my stovetop relatively low, especially when cooking with oils.

While using PUFA oils for cooking or baking is not recommended given how readily they oxidize (turn rancid), studies have shown that baking with whole or ground seeds is not nearly as destructive and actually preserves most of the ALA and other compounds.[11] (Continue reading to learn more about ALA and other essential fatty acids.) Still, I try to consume heated seeds only in moderation.

A WORD ON INDUSTRIAL OILS

The production of industrial seed oils requires the use of chemical solvents or high temperatures to extract the oil from the seeds. Canola oil, soybean oil, corn oil, and other so-called "vegetable oils" are all examples. Not only are these oils really high in inflammatory omega-6 fatty acids, but the processing strips out many beneficial nutrients. I tend to avoid these oils when cooking, opting instead for cold-pressed oils like olive or coconut that retain more of their nutritional value and have lower amounts of omega-6 fatty acids.

---

† Because of their slow oxidation rate, saturated fats can withstand longer periods of storage. So, if you're stocking a bunker, coconut oil might be a solid (eh?) addition. Food for thought.

Essential Fatty Acids

Essential fatty acids are fats that are necessary for our health. Our bodies cannot synthesize them, so we must acquire them from food or supplements. The two types of fatty acids that are essential for humans are omega-3 and omega-6 fatty acids. Because omega-3 fatty acids are found most abundantly in fish, vegans tend not to consume sufficient levels.[12]

There are a few concerns with omega-3 fatty acid deficiency in vegans, including the potential for depression as well as neurodegeneration later in life.[13] While the solution seems to be as simple as "take an omega-3 supplement," that's not really the full story here.

Balancing Omega-3 and Omega-6 Fatty Acids. To simplify things, I'm going to say that omega-6 fatty acids are typically inflammatory, while omega-3 fatty acids are anti-inflammatory. It's important to note that not all inflammation in the body is bad. When you have an injury, inflammation is the body's way of protecting the area. If you sprain your ankle, for example, the resulting swelling is fluid that is sent in to cushion the area, along with white blood cells. This swelling puts pressure on the nerves in the ankle, causing pain and disincentivizing use of the injured area. In this case, we want that inflammatory response, at least for a little while.

While some inflammation can be helpful in the short term, *chronic* inflammation in the body is currently considered to be the root cause of many (if not most) diseases.[14] Research has linked diets that have a high ratio of omega-6s to omega-3s with an increased prevalence of atherosclerosis, obesity, and diabetes,[15] whereas diets high in omega-3 fatty acids are linked with a decrease in the prevalence of these diseases.[16] Of course, correlation doesn't equal causation, but it's certainly food for thought.

Conventional wisdom in the nutrition and health community suggests that omega-3 and omega-6 fatty acids ideally should be consumed in a 1:1 ratio to keep inflammation in check. It is thought that the diets consumed by our pre-agricultural ancestors maintained this ratio and kept inflammation to a minimum. More moderate thinking is that a 1:3 ratio of omega-3 to omega-6 fatty acids is closer to an achievable ideal. Either way, current consumption patterns are pretty far from the mark. In fact, the average Western diet involves a ratio of omega-3s to omega-6s that is around 1:20 or even higher.[17]

The reason for this discrepancy is that omega-6 fatty acids are commonly found in soybean oil, corn oil, and industrial vegetable and seed oils, all of which are used in abundance in commercial cooking and processed foods.

Typically, those on a standard ketogenic diet rely on cold-water fish like salmon for their omega-3 fatty acid intake. Fish oil contains all three forms of omega-3 fatty acids—ALA, EPA, and DHA. Plant-based sources of omega-3 fatty acids, like flax seeds and walnuts, contain significant amounts of only ALA, which the body can convert to the other forms, but not particularly effectively.[18]

Adding another layer of complication, studies have demonstrated that ALA is converted even less readily in the presence of higher levels of linoleic acid (LA), the most common omega-6 fatty acid.[19] Some research suggests that given this fact, more important than the ratio is to minimize the consumption of omega-6 fatty acids while consuming omega-3s.

Because of the low conversion rate, supplementation with an algae-based omega-3 blend containing ALA, EPA, and DHA is recommended[20] for vegans to obtain the full spectrum of omega-3 fatty acids.

Sources of Omega-3 Fatty Acids. Omega-3 fatty acids are found in pretty much all types of plant foods. Seriously—100 grams of Brussels sprouts (about 5 medium-sized sprouts) contains a bit more than 20 percent of the recommended 1.6-gram intake of omega-3 fatty acids. And Brussels sprouts have a really favorable omega-3 to omega-6 ratio (2.33)—plenty of veggies do.[21]

Of course, there are far more efficient ways to consume omega-3 fatty acids that have a favorable omega-3 to omega-6 ratio. For instance, 1 tablespoon of ground flax seeds (7 grams) contains 1.6 grams of ALA. The following table lists sources of omega-3 fatty acids, as well as their omega-6 fatty acid content and the ratio.

FOOD	ALA/ omega-3 (g per 100g)	LA/ omega-6 (g per 100g)	Ratio of omega-3 to omega-6
Flax seeds	22.8	5.9	3.86
Flaxseed oil, cold-pressed	53.4	14.3	3.75
Chia seeds	17.8	5.8	3.06
Sacha inchi seeds	19.9	13.7	1.45
Hemp seeds, hulled	8.7	27.4	0.32
Walnuts	9.6	38.1	0.25

Source: USDA Food Composition Database

Reducing Omega-6 Fatty Acid Intake. As I mentioned earlier, reducing your consumption of omega-6 fatty acids is just as important as including omega-3-rich foods in your diet. This is something I regularly track in the Cronometer app. (For more about nutrient tracking, see page 35.)

For this reason, I strongly recommend avoiding industrial seed oils, soybean oil, and other vegetable oils, which are typically highly refined and very high in omega-6 fatty acids. These oils are commonly used in restaurant kitchens but also are found in commercial salad dressings, spreads, and other packaged food products. If you were wondering why I bother to make things like mayonnaise (page 183), buttery spread (page 187), and salad dressing (pages 184, 186, and 188) myself, this is a big part of the reason.

Many nuts and seeds, like almonds, Brazil nuts, pepitas (shelled pumpkin seeds), sesame seeds, and sunflower seeds, are also relatively high in omega-6 fatty acids. Because they are so nutrient dense, I do include these foods in my diet, but I consume them in moderation and balance them with foods that are rich in omega-3 fatty acids.

I promise, this isn't as complicated as it sounds! If it seems a bit overwhelming, I recommend that you start by working on including more omega-3-rich foods in your diet. Once you've tackled that, you can start reducing your omega-6 intake.

"Bad" Fats

While I don't really like to assign "goodness" to foods or macronutrients, there are some fats out there that are worth avoiding: artificial trans fats. These man-made fats provide rigidity to oil and are used in margarines and other food products where structure is necessary. (Minute amounts of trans fats exist naturally in foods—predominantly meat and dairy—but that's not what I'm talking about here.) They are also associated with cardiovascular disease and high LDL ("bad") cholesterol.[22]

While many countries have banned trans fats, they remain in the food production system in the United States and elsewhere. I want to be clear: trans fats offer no nutritional or health benefit and *do* pose health risks.[23]

Because manufacturers can "hide" trans fats on nutrition labels if the amount per serving is below 0.5 gram, it's important to check ingredient lists for partially hydrogenated oils. Unfortunately, there are still plenty of products out there (particularly vegan butter and cream cheese substitutes) that contain trans fats.

But Where Do You Get Your Protein?

I think this is the most common question that plant-based eaters hear, and it's one that can get a little old. The easy answer is "from everywhere." So many plant foods contain significant amounts of protein—grains, nuts, seeds, beans, mushrooms, greens, veggies in general—that it's pretty easy for vegans to consume their daily requirement for protein without really trying.

Things do become a bit more complicated on a ketogenic diet, however. As plant foods that contain protein also contain carbohydrates (and fats!), keeping protein intake at an adequate level while also keeping carbohydrate consumption low can present a challenge. Consuming enough protein while staying in ketosis is a totally achievable feat, but doing it entirely with whole foods as opposed to supplementing with powders, bars, or mock meat products takes a little more effort.

Essential Amino Acids & Lysine

Amino acids are the "building blocks" that make up proteins. Our bodies utilize these proteins to repair and build new tissues as well as to synthesize hormones and enzymes. There are nine amino acids that are considered essential, which is to say that we have to consume them because they cannot be synthesized by our bodies.

Animal products like meat, eggs, and dairy contain a full complement of the essential amino acids in the correct proportions, so those who consume meat, eggs, and/or dairy typically do not have to worry about specific amino acids. Vegans, on the other hand, have to be a bit more diligent. Most plant foods contain all nine amino acids, though some are present in minimal quantities. Usually, amino acid intake balances out over the course of a day or two, as long as you're eating a varied diet full of lots of different types of foods.

Older ways of thinking about vegan diets held that food combining (for example, eating beans and grains together) was the only way to consume amino acids in the proper ratio. Fortunately, this has since been debunked by numerous medical professionals.[24]

However, on a vegan keto diet, things are a tad more complicated with one amino acid in particular: lysine. Lysine is most commonly found in beans, which for ketoers typically means soybeans. If you don't eat soy products, other low-carb plant sources of lysine include lupini beans, pea protein powder, and, to a lesser degree, pepitas. Including one serving of soy, lupini beans, or pea protein powder per day should provide enough lysine to reach the required amount (assuming that you hit your overall protein requirement).[25] Most vegan protein powder blends also provide adequate lysine, though it is worth checking the labels to be sure the powder you choose contains a complete complement of amino acids in the correct ratio. Quality protein powders typically list the percentages of each amino acid present in the powder in relation to the amount the body needs.

Protein Digestibility

Another thing to be aware of when eating a vegan diet is the reduced digestibility of plant proteins. Soy and wheat proteins are generally considered to be the closest to animal proteins in terms of digestibility,[26] but for the most part, vegan proteins are simply not as bioavailable. In other words, a lower proportion of the protein present in plant foods is utilized by your body. Therefore, the general advice to vegans—especially athletes—is to err on the side of caution and consume more protein than recommended in the government's dietary guidelines.[27]

Because ketogenic diets favor moderate amounts of protein, many vegan ketoers choose to supplement with a serving of sugar-free protein powder to ensure adequate protein intake while minimizing carbohydrate consumption.

Micronutrients

In addition to macronutrients (discussed previously), it's important to keep micronutrients in mind. Micronutrients are the vitamins, minerals, and other phytochemicals that we ingest alongside the macronutrients that play crucial roles in our bodies' daily functions.

Because a ketogenic diet tends to exclude many grain products that are typically fortified with certain necessary vitamins and minerals, people who eat this way need to be aware of the potential for deficiency. Eating a balanced diet full of dark leafy greens, nuts, seeds, and other whole foods should provide adequate amounts of most micronutrients; however, a few vitamins and minerals in particular deserve additional consideration.

Be sure to talk to a healthcare professional about any supplements you are considering, especially if you have health conditions or are taking prescription medication.

Vitamin B12

The first recommendation I would make for vegans or vegetarians who don't eat eggs or dairy with any frequency is to take a vitamin B12 supplement. There is evidence that those who take metformin to treat diabetes are also at an increased risk of B12 deficiency due to reduced absorption, even if they do consume animal products.[28]

While there is some evidence that B12 can be obtained from food sources (nori and shiitake mushrooms in particular[29]), the available studies and literature are not sufficient to support this claim, so supplementation is strongly recommended.[30]

Vitamin B12 plays a crucial role in the formation of red blood cells, neurological function, and DNA synthesis,[31] as well as cardiovascular health, so it's definitely not something you want to take lightly!

There are many vegan B12 supplements available, and B12 is often included in multivitamins targeted toward vegans. You'll also note that many mock meats, nondairy milks, and other "vegan products" contain some added B12.

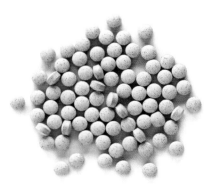

Other B Vitamins

B vitamins are commonly found in meat and fortified grain products, so those of us on a plant-based low-carb diet need to find alternative sources.

Many nuts and seeds contain sufficient B vitamins. Aside from B12, the limiting factor in vegan keto diets is often B5, or pantothenic acid. The RDA for adults is 5 milligrams,[32] which can easily be achieved with some basic planning. The following foods are good sources:

FOOD	Vitamin B5 (mg per 100g)
Sunflower seeds, raw	7.06
Shiitake mushrooms, cooked	3.59
White mushrooms, cooked	3.16
Peanuts, raw	1.77
Cremini mushrooms, raw	1.50
Avocado	1.46
Portabella mushrooms, cooked	1.26
Peanuts, roasted	1.20
Flax seeds	0.98

Source: USDA Food Composition Database

These foods all contain a spectrum of B vitamins, so I find it easier to focus on B5. Once that's in line, the rest usually are as well. Obviously, the likelihood of consuming 100 grams of flax seeds in one day is pretty low, but a medium-sized avocado actually weighs about 140 grams, so it would provide more than 40 percent of the recommended 5 milligrams of daily B5.

My favorite way to get a variety of B vitamins into my diet is to consume nutritional yeast. I like to sprinkle it on top of cooked veggies and even on avocado. It also imparts a nice "cheesy" flavor to sauces and dips. Be sure to check the label on the brand you buy; some brands are fortified with B12 and other nutrients.

Vitamin C

It might surprise you to see vitamin C listed here, but obtaining sufficient amounts of this nutrient is of some concern for those following a ketogenic diet. Vitamin C is most commonly found in fruits and vegetables and is destroyed by heat,[33] so people who are avoiding fruits and eating only small amounts of cooked veggies might find themselves deficient in this crucial vitamin.

The good news is that it's really easy to obtain enough vitamin C. The recommended daily intake for adults is 90 milligrams for men and 75 milligrams for women (this number increases to 85 milligrams for pregnant women and 120 milligrams for lactating women).[34]

To get enough vitamin C, be sure to include the following foods in your diet:

FOOD	Vitamin C (mg per 100g)
Yellow bell peppers, raw	181
Red bell peppers, raw	127
Kale, raw	93.4
Broccoli, raw	93.2
Brussels sprouts, raw	85
Broccoli, cooked	64.9
Brussels sprouts, cooked	62
Strawberries, raw	58.8
Red cabbage, raw	57

Source: USDA Food Composition Database

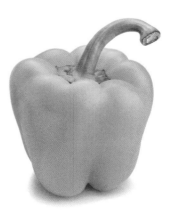

Vitamin D

Vitamin D is unique in that our bodies can produce it in response to UV exposure. Unfortunately, for a good portion of the year, most of us are tilted too far away from the sun for this process to occur. So, unless you live near the equator, chances are that for many months of the year, you aren't getting enough vitamin D. Studies also have suggested that vegans in particular are vulnerable to vitamin D deficiency.[35, 36]

Why is this important? Great question. You've likely heard that vitamin D can help your bones absorb calcium, but this fat-soluble vitamin is proving to be far more important than was once thought.[37] Recent research has suggested that vitamin D also plays a critical role in immune response and regulation, brain health, cardiovascular function, and even insulin regulation.[38]

While some quantities of vitamin D are available in mushrooms[39] and seaweed and smaller amounts are found in other plant sources,[40] vegan diets tend to be deficient in this critical nutrient, so supplementation is strongly recommended.[41]

Calcium

Most of us know that calcium plays an important role in building strong and healthy bones, but this mineral's functions extend far beyond skeletal strength. Calcium is also responsible for vascular contractions and dilations as well as hormone secretions and nerve transmissions, among other functions,[42] so obtaining a sufficient amount of this mineral is pretty important.

It is certainly *possible* for those on a plant-based diet to obtain the recommended daily allowance of calcium from whole foods alone, but it is definitely a challenge. The following chart lists ten great low-carb foods that boast a hearty amount of calcium.

FOOD	CALCIUM (mg per 100g)
Tahini	426
Almonds	265
Flax seeds	255
Collards, raw	232
Dandelion greens	187
Basil	177
Arugula	160
Brazil nuts	160
Kale, raw	150

Source: USDA Food Composition Database

While it's unlikely that anyone would eat 100 grams of tahini, almonds, or flax seeds in one day, 100 grams of greens is just a little over 3 cups and is certainly achievable. An ounce or two of other high-calcium foods on this list can also provide the necessary 1,000 milligrams of calcium.

However, this definitely takes a lot of planning, and it isn't necessarily practical on a daily basis. I love greens, and even I'm not ready to commit to eating 300 grams per day, coated in tahini and flax seeds. To make things a little easier on myself, I tend to seek out nondairy milks that are fortified with calcium, which provides about 45 percent of my daily calcium intake. The rest I can get from whole-food sources.

You could also buy a calcium supplement or look for a multivitamin specifically formulated for vegans, which will have calcium in it. Electrolyte powders and drink mixes also are sources of small amounts of calcium, as are some mineral waters.

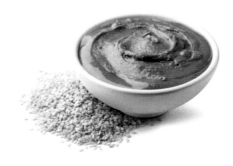

Iodine

Iodine probably isn't something you think about on a regular basis, but it's definitely worth checking in on, especially if you don't use iodized salt. (Neither sea salt nor pink Himalayan salt contains iodine.) Iodine is a crucial component in the production of thyroid hormones and thus is essential for the proper function of this gland and your metabolism.[43]

The recommended daily intake of iodine for adults is 150 micrograms, which is easily obtainable from seaweed. In fact, there have been reports of overconsumption of iodine by vegans who regularly eat seaweed.[44] Kelp added to foods (be sure to check the labels for iodine quantities) could be a sufficient source of iodine. However, the question of heavy metal contamination arises when sea vegetables come into play.

The simplest way to get adequate amounts of iodine without worrying about excess consumption or heavy metal contamination is to take a supplement. Many vegan multivitamins contain sufficient iodine.

Iron

If you've been vegan or vegetarian for a significant length of time, you're probably aware of the need to seek out foods containing iron. The approach for iron isn't that different on a ketogenic diet, though some familiar sources, like lentils, potatoes, and prunes, aren't really in play.

The recommended daily intake of iron for adults is 8 milligrams for men and 18 milligrams for women.[45] Because non-heme (plant-based) iron is less bioavailable that heme (animal-based) iron, the general recommendation for vegans and vegetarians is to increase iron consumption to 12 milligrams for men and 33 milligrams for women.[46]

The following table lists foods that are good sources of iron, though this mineral is found in other foods as well, notably dark leafy greens and olives.

FOOD	IRON (mg per 100g)
Tahini	8.95
Pepitas (pumpkin seeds), raw	8.07
Hemp seeds, hulled	7.95
Chia seeds	7.72
Sunflower seeds, raw	6.36
Flax seeds	5.73
Tofu	5.36
Hazelnuts, raw	4.70
Peanuts, raw	4.58

Source: USDA Food Composition Database

There are plenty of plant-based iron supplements available, and iron is almost always included in supplements targeted toward vegans.

Magnesium

Like potassium, magnesium is an electrolyte and is necessary for quite a few interactions within the body (more than 300 of them![47]), including muscle and nerve function, protein synthesis, and blood sugar control.

The recommended daily intake for adults is 400 milligrams for men and 310 milligrams for women, with those numbers increasing to 420 and 320 milligrams, respectively, for people over the age of fifty. These targets are easily obtainable through a whole-foods vegan keto diet without supplementation. The following chart lists the top sources of magnesium from readily available low-carb plant sources:

FOOD	MAGNESIUM (mg per 100g)
Hemp seeds, hulled	700
Pepitas (pumpkin seeds), raw	592
Cocoa powder	499
Flax seeds	392
Brazil nuts, raw	376
Tahini	362
Sunflower seeds, raw	355
Chia seeds	335
Chocolate, unsweetened	327
Almonds, roasted	279

Source: USDA Food Composition Database

While it's unlikely that anyone would eat 100 grams of any one of these foods in a single day, consuming just one 3-tablespoon (30-gram) serving of hemp seeds provides 210 milligrams of magnesium. The rest can easily be obtained by eating other seeds, nuts, and/or greens throughout the day.

Magnesium is also available as a supplement (on its own or in combination with calcium) and in electrolyte powders and mineral waters, should you and your primary care physician deem that you need more magnesium.

Potassium

Potassium also falls into the category of electrolytes, and it is critical for fluid regulation within cells.[48] (Anyone remember sodium-potassium pumps from high school biology class?) The adequate intake for potassium is listed as 4,700 milligrams per day for adult men and women.[49]

Fortunately, potassium is abundant in plant foods. The following chart lists some common low-carb plant sources of potassium:

FOOD	POTASSIUM (mg per 100g)
Hemp seeds, hulled	1,200
Beet greens, cooked	909
Sunflower seeds, dry-roasted	850
Flax seeds	813
Pepitas (pumpkin seeds), dry-roasted	809
Hazelnuts, dry-roasted	755
Almonds, raw	733
Soybeans, green, raw	620
Tahini	582
Spinach, raw	558

Source: USDA Food Composition Database

While these foods have the most potassium by weight, you can obtain this nutrient from almost all foods. Even brewed coffee has 116 milligrams of potassium in an 8-ounce (240-milliliter) cup! You can obtain smaller quantities from electrolyte powders and drink mixes as well.

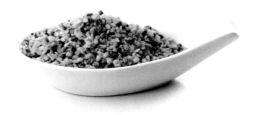

Zinc

Zinc is another nutrient that is critical to immune function. It is easily obtainable in sufficient quantities from food sources on a vegan keto diet. The RDA for zinc is 11 milligrams for men and 8 milligrams for women.[50] Because of the low bioavailability of zinc from plant-based sources, some medical professionals recommend that vegetarians and vegans increase their intake by about 30 percent.[51]

The following table provides the quantities of zinc found in 100 grams (3½ ounces) of common vegan keto foods:

FOOD	ZINC (mg per 100g)
Tahini	10.45
Pepitas (pumpkin seeds)	10.30
Sesame seeds	10.23
Hemp hearts, hulled	9.90
Cashews	5.78
Sunflower seeds	5.30
Soybeans	4.89
Chia seeds	4.53
Pecans	4.53
Almonds	3.31

Source: USDA Food Composition Database

While you are unlikely to consume this quantity of any one of these foods, you can see how easy it is to consume the recommended amount of zinc by eating one serving each of several of these foods daily.

Keeping Supplementation Simple

I like the adage, "The best *[insert thing here]* is the one you can stick to," and I definitely apply that philosophy to my supplement routine. If you think the idea of taking five pills three times a day sounds awful, I agree. I can barely remember to take my D and B12 daily!

If you know that you aren't obtaining enough nutrients from food, the easiest solution is to find a multivitamin targeted toward vegans. This should help cover the basics. You can always adjust your routine later.

Over the years, I've made a lot of changes to my supplement routine. When I worked at a health food store, I was always checking out the supplement section to see what was new and different, and my regimen was expensive and a little cumbersome. Whenever I traveled, I brought baggies and containers of pills and powders with me. It seemed totally normal then, but seems a little bit nuts to me now.

My current routine is a lot simpler. I mostly just eat a variety of foods, take algae-based omega-3, D, and B12 supplements, and add a multivitamin to the mix on some days when I'm a little low on too many nutrients. I also add a serving of sugar-free electrolyte powder to a glass of water after I work out to replenish what I lost through sweating.

My point is that you don't have to have a super-complicated supplement regimen that costs a small fortune each month. Just make sure you're giving your body what it needs!

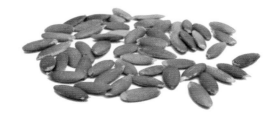

Common Keto Questions

Ketogenic and low-carb diets can be overwhelming at first. There are so many new words and concepts to learn about, not to mention the fact that keto tends to be the exact opposite of the way we have been taught to eat. It definitely takes a little time to get used to.

In the interest of making this transition easier for you, I thought I'd start off by answering some of the questions that are frequently sent my way.

Why Try Keto?

Ketogenic diets are receiving quite a bit of attention for their weight loss benefits. However, there are plenty of other reasons to consider talking to your doctor about keto. Ketogenic diets are also used therapeutically in the management and treatment of a spectrum of disorders and diseases, including diabetes, polycystic ovarian syndrome (PCOS), nonalcoholic fatty liver disease, Alzheimer's, Parkinson's, narcolepsy, depression, and cancer,[52] to name just a few.

Further research is being done on the benefits of ketosis for endocrine disorders,[53] chronic pain,[54] and even mitochondrial disorders.[55] Because of the anti-inflammatory nature of ketogenic diets, new research is revealing additional benefits each year.

How Does a Plant-Based, Vegetarian, or Vegan Keto Diet Differ from Standard Keto?

The most obvious answer is that plant-based, vegetarian, and vegan ketoers choose to omit meat, fish, bone broth, and gelatin from their diets. Those following a vegan keto way of eating also avoid eggs and dairy, as do some vegetarians and plant-based ketoers, depending on their dietary needs or concerns.

Instead of obtaining fat and protein from animal sources and consuming vegetables on the side, a plant-based model of keto focuses on consuming low-carb vegetables and obtaining fats from plant sources like nuts, seeds, coconut, olives, and avocados. Protein can be obtained from these same sources, as well as from beans. As with a standard ketogenic diet, some individuals choose to consume protein in the form of powders or bars for a convenient breakfast or snack.

Because of the increased focus on eating plant foods, which contain carbohydrates along with protein and fat, those following a vegan ketogenic way of eating often set their carbohydrate targets a bit higher than those following a conventional keto diet. This is especially true for those who follow a whole-foods vegan keto diet and choose to avoid protein powders and processed meats. (For more on determining your carbohydrate goal, check out pages 27 and 28.)

Increased vegetable consumption also tends to mean that vegans following a ketogenic diet have a higher fiber intake and often do not experience constipation when transitioning to keto.

The final main difference between vegan keto and regular keto is that vegans have to pay a little more attention to what we eat to make sure we're getting all the vitamins, minerals, amino acids, and fats our bodies need. But this isn't too different from a standard vegan diet!

Can I Do Keto Without Losing Weight?

For those whose goals don't involve weight loss, concerns can arise from seeing so many people lose weight rapidly on keto. Fear not! While water loss will cause you to drop a few pounds in the beginning, as long as you are eating enough calories, you won't continue to lose weight.

If you find that you are losing weight when you don't want to, try increasing your caloric intake. You may have to be diligent about tracking your calories (see pages 28 and 29 to learn more about tracking) to be sure you are eating enough, because a common side effect of ketosis is a reduced or suppressed appetite.

If you are trying a ketogenic diet for reasons other than weight loss, starting by eating closer to 50 grams of net carbs per day—the higher end of the recommended 20- to 50-gram range (see pages 27 and 28)—can help you enter ketosis more gently. It can also help limit the effects of the keto flu, which is covered on pages 40 and 41.

If you are following keto without weight loss as a goal, you might choose not to track in favor of a more intuitive approach, which is often called "lazy keto." Read more about intuitive eating and lazy keto on page 36.

Can I Do Vegan Keto Without Eating Soy?

The million-dollar question! Soy consumption is a pretty controversial topic in the health space, especially among vegans and vegetarians. On the one hand, soy is a great low-carbohydrate source of complete protein,[56] but it is also high in phytoestrogens, the safety of which is still under heavy debate[57] (especially for those with hormonal conditions). Additionally, many people have soy allergies and intolerances that make including this legume in their diets either extremely uncomfortable or impossible.

Whatever your reason for not wanting to consume soy, you don't have to worry—soy is definitely not a necessary component of a vegan keto diet.

I personally place soy in the "in moderation" category; I choose to indulge in some tempeh or tofu on occasion, but I don't make soy products a regular part of my diet. When I do consume soy, I try to choose those products that are the least processed (like whole edamame, tofu, and tempeh) and prioritize buying organic versions.

Most of the recipes in this book are entirely soy-free, and most that do contain soy offer simple substitutions, such as using coconut aminos in place of tamari.

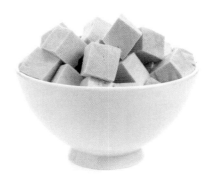

Where Is All the Gluten?

If you are gluten intolerant, I've got some good news for you! Every recipe in this book is gluten-free. I too fall into the gluten-does-terrible-things-to-my-digestion camp, so I have not included it in any form here. Keto is a pretty low-gluten diet to begin with, as gluten-containing grains are high in carbohydrates, so going completely gluten-free isn't too great a departure from the norm.

If you can eat gluten, it just opens up a few more doors. Seitan is a great source of vegan protein for those who can tolerate it. Additionally, there are some low-carb bread products on the market that contain hefty amounts of gluten.

What If I Can't Eat Nuts or Peanuts?

Again, fear not! Most of the recipes in this book are entirely nut- and peanut-free (peanuts are technically legumes, not nuts, despite having "nuts" in their name), and there are simple nut-free substitutions in almost all the nut-containing recipes. You can read more about these substitutions on page 57.

What Are Net Carbs?

Simply put, "net carbs" refers to the number of grams of carbohydrates in a serving of food that have a significant impact on your blood sugar. This number includes sugars and starches and excludes fiber and most sugar alcohols.

When someone on a ketogenic or other low-carb diet refers to daily carbohydrate intake, that person is probably referring to net carbs. In this book, when I discuss daily carbohydrate targets, I am referring to net carbs.

In the United States and Canada, the number of net carbs can be found by taking the number of grams of total carbohydrates listed on a product's nutrition label and subtracting the grams of fiber and sugar alcohols. So, for example, if a protein bar has 17 grams of total carbohydrates, 9 grams of fiber, and 6 grams of sugar alcohols, then you would count it as 2 grams of net carbs:

17 – 9 – 6 = 2 grams

In the European Union, Australia, New Zealand, and Mexico, the number of grams of carbohydrates listed on a food's nutrition label already takes fiber into account, so it doesn't need to be subtracted. Sugar alcohols still need to be subtracted, though. So that same protein bar would have a starting carbohydrate amount of 8 grams, and from that, only the 6 grams of sugar alcohols would be subtracted, for the same total of 2 grams of net carbs:

8 – 6 = 2 grams

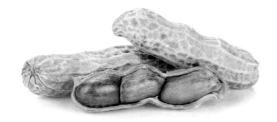

How Many Net Carbs Should I Eat?

Most people can achieve and stay in ketosis by eating between 20 and 50 grams of net carbs per day. Within this range, your personal target really depends on a few factors, including how well your body processes carbohydrates, your activity level, and your goals. There are a few different methods you can use to determine the number of grams of daily net carbs that feels best to you.

Keep in mind that this number can vary over time due to hormonal fluctuations (especially in women) and changes in your lifestyle or physical activity level, so it's worth re-evaluating how you feel periodically and increasing or decreasing your carbohydrate intake accordingly.

Choose a Starting Number Based on Your Primary Goal

I considered calling this method "determining your daily carbohydrate intake by picking an arbitrary number," because that's pretty much what it is. It's not precise or scientific, but it's the easiest way to get started.

The general idea is to pick a number between 20 and 50 grams of net carbs per day and run with it. Of course, you can tweak this number later, based on how you feel and the results you are seeing (or not seeing).

If your goal is weight loss, then choosing a target of around 20 to 35 grams of net carbs per day will help you achieve that goal faster. However, if you are beginning a ketogenic diet for other reasons, then starting out at between 40 and 50 grams is totally fine.

Determine Your Daily Carbohydrate Intake by Finding Your Carbohydrate Tolerance

This method takes a little more work, but it will help you figure out your ideal carbohydrate intake. I like this approach because it's a little more accurate. Because of the effort involved, though, it might be something to try after you are fat-adapted.

Basically, your carbohydrate tolerance is the maximum amount of carbohydrates you can eat in a day while maintaining ketosis. This is a helpful number to know if you're a big fan of eating veggies (or berries!) and want to eat as many as possible on keto. Once you've been in ketosis for a while, it is nice to know what your upper limit is.

The easiest way to check your carbohydrate tolerance is to get into ketosis and then increase your daily net carb intake by 5 grams at a time. Stay at this new level for around three days before adding another 5 grams. Once you get bumped out of ketosis (you can tell for sure by testing your ketone levels, as explained on pages 37 and 38), you know you've hit your limit and should stay closer to the previous level at which you were consistently in ketosis.

For example, say you start at 25 grams of net carbs per day. Once you hit ketosis, you would increase that number to 30 grams for three days, then 35 grams, then 40 grams, and so on until you get knocked out of ketosis. Let's say that at 50 grams per day, you are no longer in ketosis, so you would know to try to stay under 45 grams of net carbs per day.

What About That 20-Gram Number?

Twenty grams of net carbs per day has become a sort of standard in the keto community. A major reason for this is that 20 grams is a carb threshold that can help pretty much anyone reach ketosis. Another reason is that a pretty famous low-carb diet used 20 grams of net carbs as a daily limit for its "induction phase." This number is not the be-all, end-all of ketogenic diets, though! As

I've said, most individuals can reach ketosis by eating between 20 and 50 grams of net carbs per day.

The one thing that is a little challenging about limiting a vegan diet to 20 grams of net carbs per day is getting enough protein. If you compare the macronutrient breakdowns of vegan protein sources like nuts, seeds, and beans to those of animal protein sources like meat, dairy, and eggs, you'll notice one thing pretty quickly—while most of the animal sources contain very few, if any, carbohydrates, this is not the case for the plant foods. Whole-food vegan protein sources come packaged with fats and carbohydrates.

That's not to say it's an impossible task by any stretch of the imagination—plenty of foods, like hemp seeds, pepitas (pumpkin seeds), and soybeans, contain hearty amounts of protein but relatively few grams of net carbs. With careful planning, you can definitely obtain enough protein and other nutrients while keeping your carbs super low. And if you are planning on incorporating protein powders and/or mock meats into your diet, then 20 grams is a completely achievable limit.

Of course, just because you *can* keep carbs very low on a vegan keto diet doesn't mean that you have to. Whatever works best for you within the range of 20 to 50 grams is what you should stick with.

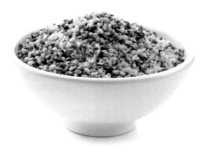

How Many Calories Should I Eat?

Before I start talking about calories, I want to hop on my soapbox and mention that I don't consider calorie intake to be quite as important as the dieting industry would have us believe. I don't mean that calories don't matter, but rather that our bodies' demands are not quite as cut-and-dried as online calculators imply.

Our needs change daily based on our activity levels, among other factors, so it's important to listen to your body's cues. If you feel extra hungry one day and go over the calorie goal you set for yourself, don't panic! Just focus on making healthy food choices and providing your body with the nutrition it needs.

Okay . . . but How Many Calories Should I Eat?

Like your carbohydrate goal, your caloric needs are determined by a constellation of factors. Online macronutrient calculators take some of these factors into account to give you a calorie target based on the number of calories you burn every day and your weight loss goal. I have a calculator on my site (http:// meatfreeketo.com/vegan-keto-macro-calculator/) to help you determine calories and macros. You can also use the built-in calculators found in many weight loss and food tracking apps.

For the greatest chance at long-term success, I recommend finding a calorie goal that is reasonable for you to maintain for extended periods. While you may be tempted to reduce your calories significantly to see quicker results, extreme caloric restriction can lead to binges.

While the calories in, calories out (CICO) model isn't perfect and isn't necessarily helpful for everyone, it's not a bad starting place if that's the model you are most comfortable with.

To figure out the average number of calories you should eat, you will want to know two important abbreviations:

- Your **Basal Metabolic Rate, or BMR,** refers to the number of calories your body requires to perform basic daily functions. I don't ever suggest eating under your BMR.

  BMR can be calculated by using several formulas. My favorite is the Katch-McArdle equation, which takes into account your lean body mass (metabolically active tissue) to determine your caloric needs. The formula is as follows:

  $$\boxed{\text{BMR}} = 370 + \left(21.6 \times \frac{\text{lean body mass}}{\text{in kilograms}} \right)$$

  If you don't know your lean body mass, use this formula to calculate it:

  $$\boxed{\substack{\text{lean} \\ \text{body} \\ \text{mass}}} = \left(\frac{\text{weight in}}{\text{kilograms}} \times 100 - \frac{\text{body fat}}{\text{percentage}} \right) / 100$$

  You can also find BMR calculators online.

- Your **Total Daily Energy Expenditure, or TDEE,** is your BMR plus the energy you burn doing everyday activities—everything from cleaning the house to walking the dog to working out at the gym. This number can be obtained from many nutrition calculators as well, and it is a rough approximation of how many calories you burn in a day.

If you are simply looking to eat fewer calories than you burn, you'll want to eat fewer calories than your TDEE, but more than your BMR. I think a reasonable caloric deficit is between 10 and 15 percent. So, if your TDEE is 2,000 calories, you want to eat between 1,700 and 1,800 calories.

Again, it's worth stating that I don't think CICO is an ideal model, but it works for many people. If you aren't one of them, don't worry—instead of focusing on calories, focus on macros or just on making healthy low-carb food choices.

How Long Does It Take to Get into Ketosis?

Exactly how long it takes to get into ketosis varies depending on your activity level, your metabolism, and how many net carbs you eat per day, but it generally takes two to three days. If you are very active, you can definitely get into ketosis within one to two days.

Keep in mind that everyone is different, so there's no need to panic if you aren't in ketosis after three days!

To find out if you are in ketosis, you can test your ketone levels. Find out how on pages 37 and 38.

What Happens If I Go Over My Carb Limit?

It is easy to exceed your carbohydrate goal, especially when you are first starting out on a ketogenic diet. I get so many messages from people saying that they started keto but went over their carb targets a few times and felt like they failed.

The first thing to remember is not to stress! It's easy to fall into the pattern of thinking you've "ruined" a day by having a few too many carbohydrates.

If you go over your carbohydrate goal by just a few grams, likely nothing at all will happen. Remember, the range for ketosis for most people is between 20 and 50 grams of net carbs per day. If you exceed your limit by a significant amount, then you might get kicked out of ketosis, but it's not a huge deal. Just keep making healthy food choices and sticking to lower-carb options, and you'll be back in ketosis before you know it!

A common phrase in the keto community is "keep calm and keto on," and I think that's especially important to keep in mind when you've gone over your carb goal and feel like you've taken a step backward.

Can I Exercise on Keto?

A big concern for many people starting out on a ketogenic diet is whether or not they'll be able to exercise. The answer is a bit complicated (surprise!). Yes, you can certainly exercise on keto—assuming that you are healthy enough to exercise, of course. (This is another conversation to have with your primary care physician!) The quality of your workouts might change, though.

When I first started keto, my primary motivation was to lose weight. So, because my friends and I had just moved into an apartment complex with a really nice gym, I thought I'd take advantage and add some cardio to my newfound diet regimen.

It did not go well. I got winded quickly and was completely defeated by the treadmill. I felt like I was running in water, so I gave up. I tried again the next day and ended up having the same experience. This lasted for several weeks.

From the messages I receive from all of you, I know I'm not alone in this. So many of you report having terrible workouts at the start of keto. The good news is that this is totally normal and will go away in time.

Studies have shown that athletes who switch to a low-carb, high-fat diet could see an overall increase in performance, but it may take the body a few weeks to several months to properly adapt to burning fat instead of glycogen.[58] In addition to enhanced performance, ketogenic diets have been shown to increase fat metabolism and decrease muscle damage during moderate-intensity exercise.[59]

Some athletes report needing a carb re-feed (see the following section for details) every five or six days to maintain performance, and others prefer to consume a slightly higher-carb protein shake or meal before a workout. Everyone reacts differently, so you may have to do some experimenting to figure out what works best for you.

While there aren't a ton of studies out there on the impact of a ketogenic diet on exercise, more research is currently underway, and I think it's a really interesting field to watch.

When Can I Have a Cheat Day or Carb Re-feed Day?

Cheat days, cheat meals, and carb re-feeds are a hot topic among people following low-carb and ketogenic diets. While cheat days/meals and carb re-feeds are a bit different, they essentially fulfill the same function, so I'm going to discuss them together.

I'll say it right from the start—I don't love using the word *cheat* to describe a higher-carb meal or day of eating. I feel that this term attaches some level of morality to a way of eating and adds an extra layer of guilt. Instead, I prefer to call "cheat days" what they really are: *higher-carb days.*

It may seem like a silly distinction, but I found that reframing the concept of a cheat day in my mind helped me have a healthier relationship with food. Calling it a "cheat day" seems to encourage bingeing for bingeing's sake. Reframing cheat days as "higher-carb

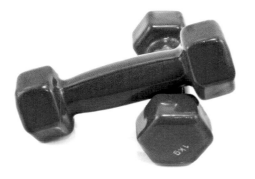

days" imparts less of a frantic need to indulge in every snack you miss from the junk food aisle of the grocery store and encourages you to think more about the nutritional aspect of those additional carbs.

Cheat Days

Basically, a cheat day is a day that you set aside for eating non-keto foods. The reason is up to you—maybe it's your birthday and you really want cake, or maybe you're just craving french fries and beer. Typically, the foods consumed on a cheat day fall into the junk food category. Cheat days also tend to involve overeating and are rooted in a desire to enjoy "forbidden" foods. The amount of carbohydrates consumed on a cheat day varies from person to person, but the driving idea is that a cheat day provides a sanctioned bacchanalian respite from the self-imposed carbohydrate asceticism that is keto.

This concept of a cheat day works really well for some people, and they're otherwise able to abstain from high-carb and sugary foods, sustained by the promise of this upcoming sugar-fest. These same people are often able to bounce back from a higher-carb day pretty quickly. Higher-carb days also help some people stay on track by providing motivation to keep eating low-carb. Knowing that you can eat some higher-carb foods on a predetermined day might keep you eating low-carb the rest of the time without bingeing on chips or candy. If this system works for you, then go for it.

When you plan for a higher-carb day (or single meal) is really up to you, though I don't recommend it within the first three to four weeks after switching to keto. Give yourself time to adjust to the diet before adding in any more complications. After that, some people like to have a cheat day or meal once a week, while others find that once a month works better—and some never have cheat days at all. It all depends on how higher-carb days make you feel.

Carb Re-feeds

Carb re-feed days tend to serve a more practical purpose. Certain people, like athletes and some women, just need more carbs to feel good, but they still want to experience the benefits of ketosis. Carb re-feed days provide a solution. Some people report feeling much better if they have a carb re-feed once a week or so, including endurance and physique athletes.[60]

Typically, carb re-feed days are scheduled, occurring once a week or so, and focus on consuming carbohydrates in a controlled way. Instead of unlimited pizza or ice cream, a carb re-feed day might involve eating a cup of rice or sweet potato with lunch and dinner in order to replenish glycogen stores in the body. (Refer to pages 8 and 9 for more on glycogen stores.) Fat intake tends to be lower on carb re-feed days to mitigate unwanted weight gain. Some people limit their fat intake to 50 grams on these days.

When you schedule a carb re-feed is entirely up to you. Again, I wouldn't recommend it within the first three to four weeks of switching to keto, as your body will still be adjusting to a low-carb diet. However, if you notice that after a month or so, you are feeling tired and sluggish and a little worn out, you might want to try a carb re-feed to see if it helps you.

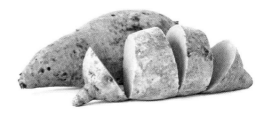

Maintenance & Beyond!

Once you hit your weight loss goal, you can begin what's known as the maintenance phase of keto. In this phase, you might choose to remain in ketosis for the other benefits it provides, but you don't want to continue losing weight.

The maintenance phase typically involves increasing both your caloric intake and your net carbohydrate intake so that you maintain your current weight. In maintenance, you tend to have a little more freedom with what you eat; many people choose to stop tracking at this point and eat more intuitively. (Read more about intuitive eating and "lazy keto" on page 36.)

If you want to remain in ketosis, it's a good idea to find out your carbohydrate tolerance (see pages 27 and 28), especially if you wish to incorporate more veggies or fruits into your diet.

For some people, maintenance might mean eating a typical low-carb (but not ketogenic) diet of between 50 and 150 grams of net carbs per day and eating more starches and fruit. If this approach feels best for your body, then go for it! The important thing is to find out what is most sustainable for you.

For me, maintenance means eating what I want when I want. I choose to eat lower-carb foods, so most of the time I am in a state of ketosis. There are times, though, when I'll kick myself out of ketosis by eating higher-carb foods. I don't worry so much anymore about whether I'm "eating keto"; I just focus on eating anti-inflammatory, nutrient-dense whole foods for most of my meals and making sure I'm providing my body with the necessary micronutrients.

What Do You Eat in a Day?

Many of the questions that pop up frequently in my inbox revolve around how I personally eat and what keto looks like long-term. It's been six years since I started a plant-based ketogenic way of eating, and over the years, what I eat in a day has changed a lot.

Now that I am in maintenance mode, I don't tend to worry about keeping my carbs super low. Nor do I tend to stress about calories. I aim to eat between 30 and 50 grams of net carbs (with the bulk of those carbs coming from veggies and some berries) and between 2,000 and 2,200 calories on a daily basis. Of course, on some days I eat more than 2,200 calories, and on other days I eat barely 1,600. I just try to eat when I'm hungry, stop eating when I'm full, and make food choices that will make my body feel good.

As far as the actual foods I eat, I usually have coffee or a Coconut Matcha Latte (page 158) in the morning. For "breakfast," whenever that might happen, I usually have some variation on Avocado Toast (page 76) or "Noatmeal" (page 65) with a green smoothie. Lunch is almost always a giant salad with lots of greens and some crunchy veggies. Dinner changes all the time, depending on what recipe I'm working on for my blog. A pretty typical snack for me is peanut butter out of the jar with a spoon. I'm not even remotely kidding.

To get a general idea of the types of meals I eat, just check out the recipes in this book! These recipes are very representative of my typical eating habits. I also write the occasional "What I Eat in a Day" post on my blog, and you can find all those posts here: http://meatfreeketo.com/category/what-i-eat-in-a-day/

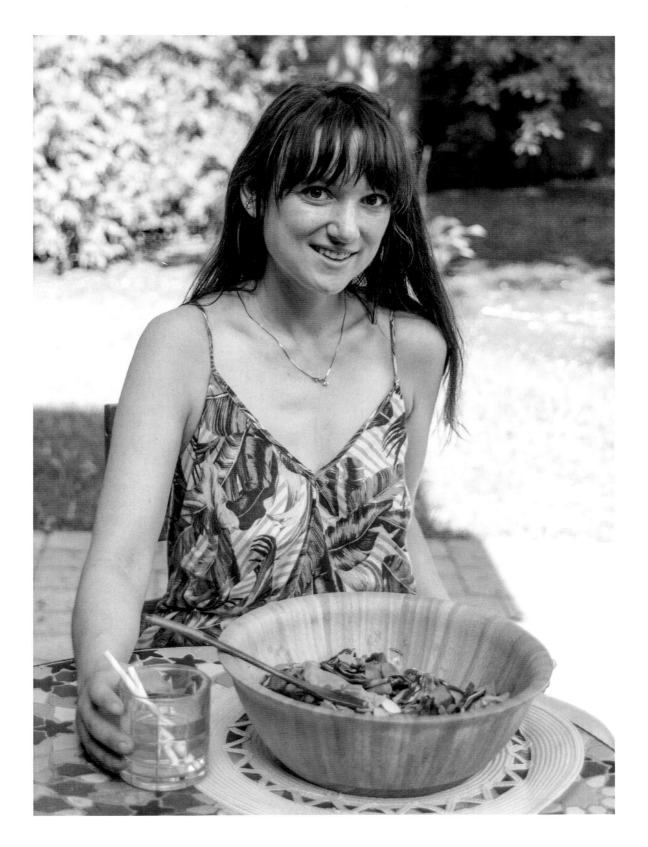

How to Get Started on a Ketogenic Diet

Now that you know what a ketogenic diet is, let's talk about how to get started! Like anything else, you can make keto as simple or as complicated as you want. Not everyone is comfortable with weighing out and writing down every bit of food that goes into their mouth, and by the same token, not everyone feels confident in making food choices without having some guidelines to follow.

Fortunately, you can tailor your approach by using one of the two main styles of keto dieting: tracking and lazy keto. You can use either method or switch between them as you like. I often combine the two—taking a lazy keto approach to which foods I choose to eat and then retroactively tracking them because I love analyzing information.

This has definitely changed over time. When I first started out on keto, I kept track of only net carbs to make things as easy as possible for myself. A few weeks in, I began to track other macronutrients as well. After five or six months, I stopped tracking and embraced a lazy keto approach, and then, as I started blogging more frequently and creating meal plans, I got serious about my tracking game and started looking at both macronutrients and micronutrients.

There is no need to tie yourself to one method over the other. Try out both approaches to see which works better for you!

Tracking

If you're a person who loves data, then boy, do I have good news for you! Being a way of eating that focuses on macronutrients, keto lends itself well to aggressive food tracking.

Within the realm of tracking, you can choose to focus on certain aspects (for example, macronutrient ratios or net carb goals) or go all out and track literally everything. There is no one right way to track what you eat.

Tracking Just Carbohydrate Intake

This is certainly the easiest approach to tracking what you eat on keto. I started out this way, and I find it to be the most user-friendly approach overall. Basically, you focus on tracking your net carbohydrate intake with the goal of keeping it under a certain limit.

In the beginning, I set 20 grams of net carbs as my goal. I kept a running tally of the carbs I consumed throughout the day without stressing about total calories, grams of protein, or percentage of fat. I did this for the first full week until I had become accustomed to this new way of eating; only then did I start to track other targets, like calories, protein, and fat. Having just one thing to worry about really helped me focus and kept keto from becoming too overwhelming.

Was I eating a super balanced diet? Probably not, but balance was something I ironed out later. I definitely recommend this style of tracking for those who want to have some sort of goal but aren't super excited about having to worry about balancing macronutrients.

You don't need to download an app for tracking your carb intake (although you can use one; see below for a list of apps); a simple notebook will do the trick. See page 36 for more on keeping a food diary.

Tracking Macronutrient Percentages

If you're ready for something a little more advanced than keeping track of net carbs, you could consider tracking your intake of total carbohydrates, protein, and fat. For this approach, I definitely recommend downloading an app like MyFitnessPal, LoseIt, or Cronometer. These apps let you set custom macronutrient goals and then give you a breakdown of how many grams of each macronutrient you should eat. Keep in mind that many apps don't have a "net carbs" setting (though Cronometer does!), so you may have to calculate that number manually.

Many people who follow a ketogenic diet like to keep their fat, protein, and carbohydrate intakes within certain ranges:

- Fat intake is typically between 60 and 80 percent of total calories.

- Protein intake is generally between 15 and 30 percent of total calories.

- Net carbohydrates are limited to 5 to 10 percent of total calories.

As you can see, you have a fairly broad range to work within these parameters.

Those on a whole-food vegan keto diet may find themselves consuming closer to 10 percent of their daily calories in carbohydrates, as nearly all sources of vegan protein also contain carbs.

You can either log your meals preemptively based on what you plan to eat that day or log after each meal. I don't recommend waiting until the end of the day to log everything in one fell swoop, as it can be hard to remember every little thing you ate or drank.

It might seem a little tedious at first to have to enter everything into an app (or a physical food diary, if your style is more analog), but after a while it becomes second nature, and writing everything down usually takes less than two minutes.

Most apps also allow you to track your body weight and measurements so you can see your progress over time.

Tracking Everything

Finally, if you're a little bored with tracking just your macronutrients, you could branch out and start obsessing over micronutrients and calories as well. Unless you're a seasoned food tracker, I would hold off here until you are quite established in a keto routine.

The website and app I recommend for tracking everything is Cronometer. The "basic" features (which are still pretty advanced!) are free and allow you to keep track of everything from vitamins and minerals to types of fat to specific amino acids. These features can be really helpful if you want to obtain as many nutrients as possible from foods instead of relying on too many supplements.

A note on tracking calories: While I do think calorie intake can be a helpful guideline for some people, there's no need to become obsessive or rigid about it. If you go over your calorie target one day, don't panic! Your body's needs fluctuate daily based on factors like hormone levels, exercise intensity, and even the amount of sleep you got the night before.

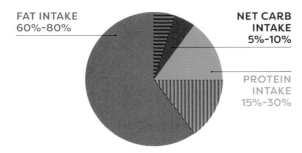

FAT INTAKE
60%-80%

NET CARB INTAKE
5%-10%

PROTEIN INTAKE
15%-30%

Lazy Keto

If tracking everything you eat in a day and trying to balance out macros and calories seems a little overwhelming, don't panic! There is another way. Often called "lazy keto," this approach basically just involves eating low-carb foods and avoiding higher-carb foods. That's it. No stress, no tracking apps, and no mental math every time you are thinking of getting a snack.

Lazy keto is great if you don't want to add an extra layer of complication to your daily routine and would rather just focus on trying to make good food choices. This approach can work really well if you aren't trying to lose weight but still want to be in ketosis.

Lazy keto is a good fit not only for beginners who are trying to get their footing, but also for pros who have been on a ketogenic diet long enough to have reached the maintenance phase. It's certainly the most sustainable way of eating, as the majority of people don't want to be tied to a calorie and macronutrient tracker for each and every meal.

I love the lazy keto approach because it allows you to focus on how your body is responding to what you're eating and make adjustments without worrying about hitting certain macronutrient or calorie targets. It gives you the opportunity to practice intuitive eating within the framework of a ketogenic diet.

Yes, upon cursory examination, these two concepts do seem to be mutually exclusive, but don't let that fool you! You can certainly practice mindfulness and apply many of the principles of intuitive eating to a ketogenic or low-carb way of eating.

- **Avoid eating while distracted by the TV or your computer.** It can be easy to overeat if you aren't really paying attention to your meal.

- **Take a moment to consider what your body is trying to tell you.** Often, thirst signals are misinterpreted as hunger. Try drinking some water when you first feel hungry. If that doesn't do the trick, then you probably are actually hungry.

- **Chew your food completely and pause between bites.**

- **Take note of how certain foods affect you.** Consider keeping a food diary to help you identify the relationships between the foods you eat and how you feel both physically and emotionally.

Keeping a Food Diary

Even if you don't track your calories or closely monitor your macronutrient intake, I think that keeping a food diary can be an incredibly valuable exercise.

When I first started studying nutrition, my advisor tasked me with keeping a seven-day food diary. I went into it feeling pretty confident that I knew what I was eating and how it was impacting me. After all, I was interested in nutrition and I was a vegan. Didn't that mean I was eating healthfully already?

As it turned out, no. No, it didn't. My diary revealed that my steady diet of pasta with frozen veggies, sugary protein bars, and coconut milk lattes was leaving me exhausted, irritable, bloated, and constantly hungry. Who knew?

I was actually kind of embarrassed when I turned in that assignment, but we all have to start somewhere, and seeing everything written out really helped me make connections between certain reactions I was having and the foods that were causing them.

Your food diary can be as simple or complicated as you want to make it. You basically want to write down the following information:

- The time of each meal or snack
- How you felt before eating
- The food(s) you ate
- How you felt immediately after eating
- How you felt about an hour after eating

How you felt could be either physical or emotional. Were you sad? Anxious? Did you experience bloating? Did you get really sleepy? All of these types of reactions are important.

You can use a notebook, a computer spreadsheet, or even the notes app on your phone. I just take notebook paper and write out a simple table like the one below whenever I'm keeping a food diary.

Note: This is how I noticed that soy doesn't wholly agree with my digestive system. It sounds silly, but sometimes you don't notice what you're not looking for. So, when I stopped and assessed how I felt immediately after eating soy and an hour later, I realized that it wasn't just gluten that my digestive system couldn't handle. Soy was a problem, too.

It's also worth noting that your body may react differently to foods under different circumstances. Every few months, you may want to do food diary entries for a week or so to see where you are with various foods, like soy, nuts, and seeds.

Ketone Testing

When I first started keto, I wanted to know if I was in ketosis all the time. I'd wake up in the morning and use a ketone test strip. I'd test again when I got home from work. I'd test at night before going to bed, just to see if anything had changed. I was so excited about keto that I wanted to quantify every second of it.

For those first few weeks, it sure was fun, but eventually, the novelty of seeing that little strip turn dark pink wore off, and I began to rely on other signs to see what was going on in my body.

While I do recommend testing at the beginning, it's not necessary to test your ketone levels all the time. If you are seeing results and feeling great, then there's really no reason to go to the expense. However, testing can be a nice way to figure out your carb tolerance and your protein tolerance and even see if certain foods kick you out of ketosis.

It's important to remember that over time, as your body becomes more efficient, it will down-regulate the production of ketones. So, while you may still be in ketosis, you may not continue to put up those high numbers like you did in the beginning. This is totally normal and shouldn't be discouraging!

Whether you are in a light state of ketosis (producing between 0.5 and 1.5 mmol/L of ketones) or a heavier state, you are still in ketosis.

Sample Food Diary Entries

TIME	FOOD EATEN	HOW I FELT			NOTES
		Before eating	Immediately after eating	1 hour after eating	
7:00 a.m.	Coffee w/ coconut milk	Tired, not yet awake	Happy, excited, energized	A little bit hungry	
9:30 a.m.	Homemade peanut butter protein bar	A little bit hungry	Satisfied	Energized	
1:00 p.m.	Salad w/ tofu and olives	Very hungry, a little tired	Full, a bit sleepy	Bloated and uncomfortable	Maybe soy caused the bloating?

"Keto Sticks"

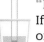

If you belong to any online keto groups or follow keto hashtags on social media, you've probably noticed a lot of pictures of ketone test strips. Often called "keto sticks," these little testers have a pad on one end that can detect ketone levels in your urine. Yes, you pee on them.

The strips turn increasingly deeper shades of pinkish purple, depending on how many ketones are detected in your urine. They're not the most accurate method, but they are relatively inexpensive and widely available; they can be purchased wherever diabetic testing supplies are sold. In the United States, this includes basically every pharmacy and the majority of grocery stores and big-box stores.

These strips can be helpful at the very beginning for providing some quantification of the degree of ketosis you are experiencing, but they don't really give you the full picture. Ketone production fluctuates throughout the day and can change depending on whether you've exercised recently or on hormonal fluctuations.

It's important to note that as you become fat-adapted, your body becomes more efficient and produces fewer ketones. So if, after a while, those test strips don't turn quite so pink, it's nothing to worry about. The results shown on the strips are also dependent on your hydration levels, so you may be showing higher ketone production because you are dehydrated. Conversely, you may show minimal or even zero ketone production if you are drinking lots of water.

PROS: Cost-effective | CONS: Not the most accurate; can give false readings due to hydration levels and degree of fat-adaptation

Ketone Breath Meter

Ketone breath meters are another tool for testing ketone production, as ketones are excreted through the breath as well as the urine. While these meters don't give you an exact reading of your current ketone production, they are able to tell you whether you are in ketosis.

PROS: Mostly accurate | CONS: Expensive

Ketone Blood Meter

If you absolutely love gathering data, a ketone blood meter is a good option for tracking your ketone levels. Most of these meters double as blood glucose monitors, so you can check both with one device. The downside to these meters is that the test strips can be pretty costly, ranging from $1 to $3 each. Another downside is that you have to prick yourself with a lancet to draw blood for each test, which is a deal breaker for some people.

On the other hand, this method of testing is quite accurate and can even help you see how certain foods affect you based on whether those foods kick you out of ketosis. Testing your blood ketone levels about an hour after eating a food you are unsure of can yield really helpful information, especially if you're dealing with a stall in your progress and want to know the culprit. Because testing your blood ketone levels after each meal can get expensive, though, I suggest holding off unless you feel it is absolutely necessary.

PROS: Accurate; also tests blood glucose levels | CONS: Expensive; requires blood drawing

CHECKING BLOOD GLUCOSE

Some people also keep track of their blood glucose levels while on a ketogenic diet. This is especially important for those who may be prediabetic, hypoglycemic, or otherwise metabolically deranged. Be sure to test your blood sugar levels at the same time each day. Note whether you are fasted or how long after a meal you are testing in order to establish a consistent pattern. Blood sugar levels are typically higher right after you wake up in the morning, so waiting an hour or so to test will give you a reading that is more representative of your typical levels.

According to the American Diabetes Association, a "normal" range for blood sugar is between 80 and 100 mg/dL. If you are worried about your blood glucose levels, you should definitely talk with your doctor.

Reading Your Body's Signs

The last way to determine whether you've entered a state of ketosis is to pay close attention to how your body feels. These signs may be hard for you to distinguish at first, but the more times you cycle in and out of ketosis (either from higher-carb days or from practicing cyclical keto—you'll find more on both of those concepts on pages 30 and 31), the more apparent they will become.

As I mentioned earlier, one of the most important benefits I have experienced on a ketogenic diet is a heightened awareness of my body and the signals it's trying to send me. While I do test my ketones occasionally out of curiosity, I have learned to notice when I'm back in ketosis based on how my body feels, using the signs discussed in this section.

Everyone reacts differently to ketosis, but these are some common effects that I (and many others in the keto community) have experienced.

Increased Thirst

One of the first signs you may notice when you are in ketosis is that you are thirstier than normal. This is because glycogen storage in the body requires water, so when you deplete those glycogen stores, your body releases this water, leading you to feel thirstier. You might have a cottony feel in your mouth, or you might simply be unusually thirsty. This feeling shouldn't last for more than a week, though.

Be aware that dramatic increases in thirst can be indicative of a health problem. If you are constantly drinking water and consuming sufficient electrolytes (see page 41) but still feel dehydrated, contact your doctor.

Changes in Urine

It might sound strange, but you should familiarize yourself with your urine. Often, changes in urine indicate that something is going on in your body healthwise, so it's nice to have an idea of what your urine is like on a typical day.

The increase in fluid consumption (associated with increased thirst) will naturally lead you to take more trips to the bathroom. This is normal at the beginning and can be a sign that you are in ketosis!

In addition to increased frequency, you may notice other changes in your urine. When you enter a state of ketosis, you excrete ketone bodies via urination.[61] These excreted ketones can give your urine a shiny, almost oily appearance. You may also notice that your urine appears lighter in color due to increased fluid consumption.

Changes in Stool

Like your urine, your stools can be a great indicator of health, so it can't hurt to give them a quick look every once in a while to check for changes.

For me, eating a low-carb diet transformed my bowel movements from erratic and crampy, with alternating bouts of loose stools and constipation, to regularly occurring, smooth, and pain-free morning (and sometimes bonus afternoon) experiences. Others with IBS share similar stories about changes in their bowel movements after they switched to a ketogenic diet.

Of course, this is not everyone's experience. Many people notice a day or two of constipation or loose stools when entering ketosis. Constipation tends to occur in individuals who are consuming less fiber on a ketogenic diet. This side effect does not seem to be as prevalent among vegans and vegetarians, who typically consume larger amounts of high-fiber foods, like nuts, seeds, and vegetables, than their meat-eating counterparts.

While one or two days of abnormal bowel movements are within the realm of what can be expected, anything beyond that is worth addressing with a healthcare professional.

Bad or Weird-Smelling Breath

Ketones are expelled from your lungs and into your mouth and the air around you when you breathe out. Therefore, when you enter ketosis, you may notice a change in how your mouth tastes and how your breath smells. Many people report a somewhat fruity scent to their breath.

Increased Mental Clarity

This is the most nebulous and difficult-to-define sign that you are in ketosis. Many people on a ketogenic diet experience a lifting of brain fog and find themselves able to think more clearly. Additionally, individuals have noted feeling sharper and more alert.

Of course, the converse can be true as well. Brain fog is a symptom of the dreaded keto flu (see below), though not everyone experiences it. Thankfully, the keto flu is temporary, and any fog should lift before too long.

Less Swelling and Inflammation

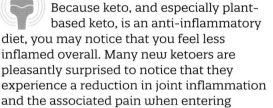

Because keto, and especially plant-based keto, is an anti-inflammatory diet, you may notice that you feel less inflamed overall. Many new ketoers are pleasantly surprised to notice that they experience a reduction in joint inflammation and the associated pain when entering ketosis.

One of the best effects of keto for me is that my joints feel nice and loose—not like they're not properly supported, but more like there isn't any resistance when I use them.

Surviving the Keto Flu

You've probably heard the phrase "keto flu," and it may have made you a bit nervous. After all, the symptoms don't sound great: fatigue, body aches, nausea, gastrointestinal trouble, irritability, brain fog, insomnia, light-headedness, muscle cramping—this is not a party I want an invite to.

Of course, not everyone gets the keto flu. While many people do experience some keto flu–related issues, others never notice anything at all. So you may never have to deal with any of the above symptoms.

However, in case you do find yourself feeling kind of blah after a few days of eating a ketogenic diet and fear that the keto flu is coming on, the following tips should bring you some relief until the symptoms pass. Symptoms typically abate within three to seven days, although some people report experiencing the keto flu for a bit longer than that.

Replenish Electrolytes— They're What You Crave

Many of the symptoms of keto flu can be attributed to dehydration. When your body first enters ketosis, you start burning up the glycogen stored in your liver and muscles. Because glycogen requires some water to be stored, once the glycogen goes, so will a lot of water. With that water will go waste products but also electrolytes that are critical for the fluid balance in your body, as well as nerve signaling and muscle function.[62]

To combat the symptoms caused by electrolyte imbalance, including fatigue, muscle cramping, light-headedness, and digestive issues such as diarrhea, make sure you're eating enough mineral-rich foods (see pages 22 and 23). If you still feel like you need more electrolytes, try drinking any of the following throughout the day:

- Mineral water
- 8 ounces (240 ml) of water mixed with 1 teaspoon of lemon juice and a pinch of salt
- Herbal tea
- Vegetable broth

Additional electrolyte consumption is especially important if you participate in a sport or other activity that makes you sweat a lot. Some people have tried drinking pickle juice throughout the day to replenish electrolytes, and while it may work for less-active individuals, pickle juice doesn't fully replenish electrolytes in athletes.[63]

Eat More Fat!

While some keto flu issues can be resolved by increasing your electrolyte intake, others are related to the fact that you are likely experiencing sugar cravings. This is the one "symptom" I dealt with while transitioning into ketosis. The main culprit behind carb cravings is the addictive nature of carb-laden processed foods.[64] Switching to a fat-based way of eating can induce sugar withdrawal.

The easy solution for me was to eat more fatty foods like avocados and macadamia nuts, even if it meant going over my calorie and/or carb target for the day. This did the trick, and within a couple of days, my appetite had normalized and I no longer wished that everything I was eating was pasta. This approach seems to have worked for many others in the keto community as well.

Get Some R & R

Keto flu symptoms also can be brought on by stress and a lack of sleep. Be kind to yourself, practice good self-care, and make sure you're sleeping enough, especially when you're first transitioning to a ketogenic diet. Similarly, try to cut down on stress wherever possible. If this means taking a half-hour walk in the woods, fantastic. If all you can manage is two minutes of meditation with an app on your phone, also fantastic.

Self-care isn't about applying every face mask you own, lying in an Epsom salt bath, and lighting scented candles while you listen to gong music. I mean, it can be, but it doesn't *have* to be. Self-care is about doing whatever you have the time or energy for to treat yourself.

Gentle movement like a walk or some light yoga can also help you feel a bit better when facing keto flu symptoms.

Tips for Starting Keto Stress-Free

Save Time in the Kitchen

Sometimes saving a few extra minutes here and there can make all the difference in the world. Thanks to the popularity of the Paleo diet, many grocery stores now offer premade cauliflower rice and zucchini noodles in the cut produce section. Having these ingredients ready to go can take some of the stress out of putting a meal together.

Buying frozen vegetables is another way to save time—all the prep work is already done for you! Plus, you can buy frozen veggies in bulk and store them for quite a while, which saves you some money, too.

Finally, while I have included recipes for spice blends, spreads, sauces, and dressings, you don't have to make them all yourself in order to succeed on a vegan ketogenic diet. There are plenty of commercially available products that don't contain added sugars and are made with quality ingredients. I tend to look at brands that target the Paleo market because Paleo puts an emphasis on ingredient quality. So, if you really don't have time to make your own mayo (the cleanup is the tough part there), store-bought mayo is more than fine.

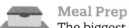

Meal Prep

The biggest thing that saves me time and makes my week go more smoothly is doing meal prep in advance, and I know I'm not alone in that. A quick search for the hashtag #MealPrepSunday shows just how many people are embracing meal prep to help with healthier eating.

For me, meal prep usually means deciding what I'm going to eat that week and then spiral-slicing the veggies and making the various condiments or sauces required for those meals—basically, the tasks that take that little bit of extra time. I'll also make up some jars of the dry ingredients for Overnight Noats (page 65) or Basic Chia Pudding (page 78) so I've got a handy breakfast option available in a pinch.

Ignore the Opinions of Strangers on the Internet

People on the internet can be really opinionated, especially when it comes to diet and fitness. Over the past few years of belonging to numerous keto and low-carb message boards and social media groups, I've seen a lot of people excitedly post their meals or screenshots of their macro charts for the day only to be immediately bombarded with unsolicited comments informing them of all the ways those meals/macros are wrong and decidedly Not Keto.

Of course, this is not true of the vast majority of keto support groups out there, but just one negative comment can really put a damper on your day. If you do choose to join a keto support group on social media, make sure to find one that is healthy, positive, and supportive. The group's dynamic should be pretty clear from the comments left on members' posts.

One of the best online communities I've found is a Facebook group called Vegan Keto Made Simple. It's run by an awesome group of really supportive and wonderful people and is definitely worth checking out.

At the end of the day, you should feel free to practice keto in whatever way feels best and healthiest to you. If someone in your keto group doesn't like that you put blueberries in your smoothie, this is his or her problem, not yours!

Don't Worry About the Little Things

Did you accidentally eat one and a half servings of almonds instead of just one? Not sure how much salad dressing you used? Were you extra hungry and couldn't help but eat a fat bomb that wasn't on your meal plan? Don't stress about it!

It's unlikely that one small deviation from your plan will derail your progress. Even if you are kicked out of ketosis temporarily, continuing to eat a ketogenic diet will put you right back into a fat-burning state.

I like to think of these situations as learning experiences more than "setbacks" or "missteps." Did you eat too many carbs today? Well, take note of how those extra carbs made you feel and store that information away for the next time you're considering a piece of cake.

Whenever you start to stress about something, such as going over your calorie or carb target or eating enough (or too much) protein in a given day, just remember—keep calm and keto on.

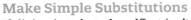

Make Simple Substitutions

If diving into keto headfirst isn't your style, there's no need to worry. Sometimes the easiest way to get started on a ketogenic diet is to take dishes you already love and simply swap out the carbohydrate-rich component for its low-carb counterpart. For instance, you can replace the rice in your favorite curry or stir-fry with cauliflower rice or the noodles in your favorite pasta dish with zucchini noodles.

By making substitutions for these higher-carb foods, you can dip your toes into low-carb and ketogenic eating without having to overhaul your diet. As you become more comfortable with eating fewer carbohydrates, you can continue to make substitutions and remove more higher-carb elements from your meals and see how you feel.

You can also try switching out one full meal per day at a time. For example, you could eat a bowl of High-Protein "Noatmeal" (page 65) for breakfast in lieu of your normal bowl of cereal. Then, the next week, you could replace your sandwich at lunch with a low-carb salad. Finally, in the third week, you could start making keto dinners for yourself as well.

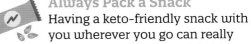

Always Pack a Snack

Having a keto-friendly snack with you wherever you go can really help you out. I like to keep nonperishable foods like trail mix and protein bars in my desk drawer, car, and purse. This way, no matter where I am, I know I have a healthy option. Packing low-carb snacks helps prevent those moments when you're just too hungry to wait any longer to eat, and vending machine cookies and pretzels are your only options.

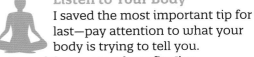

Listen to Your Body

I saved the most important tip for last—pay attention to what your body is trying to tell you.

One of the greatest benefits I've experienced on a ketogenic diet is having a better understanding of the messages my body is sending me. I've learned to pay close attention to how different foods affect how I feel and to modify how I eat accordingly. Some days you may feel like you need more protein or more fat or more calories in general. It's important to listen to your body's signals and make adjustments in response. While meal plans and macronutrient targets provide a helpful framework, they don't account for biological differences across populations, nor do they adapt to changes in our day-to-day routines.

I know I say this a lot, but it really is important to remember that we are all very different and that your personal needs can change. So, if you feel like something isn't working for you, it's worth taking a second look at it.

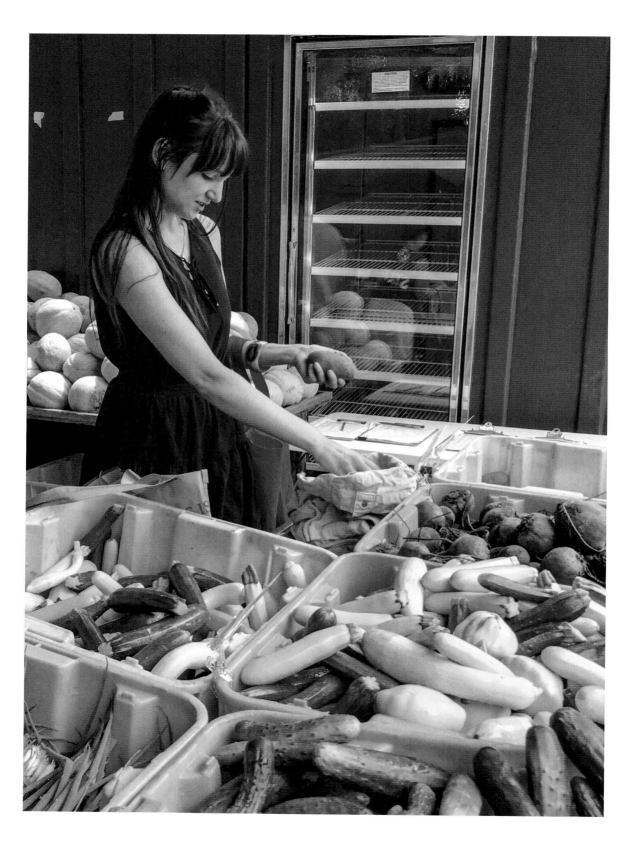

What to Eat on a Vegan Keto Diet

I've said it before and I'll say it again: there is no one "right" way to eat a ketogenic diet. As long as you are in ketosis, you are eating keto. However, there are some guidelines that can help make a ketogenic diet more nutrient dense and a little easier to follow, especially during the initial adjustment period.

Prioritize Whole Foods

I'm a huge fan of seeking out whole foods over their processed counterparts. When I talk about processing, I don't mean fermenting, blending, spiral-slicing, or otherwise changing a food in a way that you could change it in your kitchen. I'm talking about food products that are produced in a lab.

I seek out as many whole foods as possible because they tend to be more nutrient dense and also more difficult to overeat (at least in my experience!). While you can obtain vitamins and minerals from supplements, evidence suggests that the sum of the nutritional value of whole foods is greater than their constituent parts.[65] There are so many flavonoids and other beneficial phytochemicals in vegetables, fruits, nuts, seeds, and legumes that appear to work synergistically, with studies demonstrating that therapeutic use of isolated versions of those compounds is often either less effective or wholly ineffective.[66]

Additionally, though protein bars and other packaged snacks are tasty and convenient, you might hurt your chances of entering ketosis if you indulge in these types of treats too often. Many contain sweeteners that can kick you out of ketosis if consumed in excess. Plenty of ketoers have noted that some of the so-called low-carb sweeteners in these bars actually do impact blood sugar in certain people. So, while a bar might claim to have just 3 grams of net carbs, that might not be the case in reality.

The 80/20 Principle

When it comes to figuring out what to eat on a daily basis, I find the 80/20 principle really helpful. It suggests that at least 80 percent of your food choices should come from whole-food sources, with the remaining 20 percent being more on the "convenience foods" side. On a 2,000-calorie diet, this would mean roughly 1,600 calories coming from whole foods and the remaining 400 calories coming from processed sources like protein bars and powders, mock meats, and "indulgences" like alcoholic beverages. I also include keto baked goods and desserts in this category.

This isn't so much a hard-and-fast rule as it is a way to steer your food decisions. Of course, you don't need to include that 20 percent, but it's a nice guideline to have.

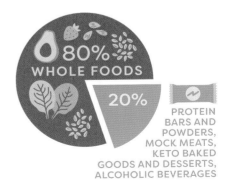

Which Foods Are Forbidden on Keto?

I mentioned this before, but I think it is a really important point to address: *there are no "forbidden" foods on keto.* A ketogenic diet is comprised of any foods that fuel your body and keep you in a state of ketosis. For most people, this means avoiding starches and grains, as well as soda and sugar-sweetened foods, because they are so high in carbohydrates that it is difficult to consume them without being kicked out of ketosis.

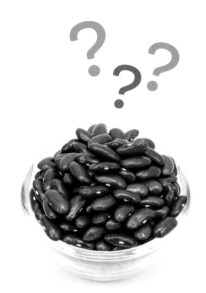

Many people also choose not to consume beans or fruit, which are higher in carbohydrates. However, this does not mean that beans and fruit are not "allowed." As long as you eat these foods in small enough quantities that you stay in ketosis, then they are perfectly suitable for a ketogenic diet. I know many keto dieters who budget their daily carbohydrate intake to include hummus because it's just so tasty that it's worth including.

INGREDIENTS TO AVOID

In addition to checking food nutrition labels for macronutrients, it can be helpful to look at the ingredients. While, as vegans, we are already pretty used to checking labels for hidden egg and dairy ingredients, there are a few other ingredients to watch out for when looking for keto-friendly foods:

• **Hydrogenated oils**—*These oils contain trans fats and are sometimes found in vegan dairy substitutes and nut butters.*

• **Sucralose, aspartame, saccharin, and other artificial sweeteners**—*Some people notice that artificial sweeteners can cause weight loss to stall and even kick them out of ketosis.*

• **Maltitol**—*This sugar alcohol causes a lot of gastrointestinal distress and spikes blood sugar to boot.*

• **Added sugars**—*While most plant-based foods (even spinach!) contain some natural sugars, added sugars are easy to avoid. Check nutrition labels for the "added sugars" line and watch out for ingredients ending in –ose. While some people have no problem eating small amounts of added sugars on a ketogenic diet, others find that even a few grams of sugar can kick them out of ketosis. Honey, maple syrup, and agave nectar also should be avoided.*

My Top Five Vegan Keto "Superfoods"

I know—the word *superfood* gets tossed around *a lot,* but there are some foods that I think more than pull their weight on a vegan keto diet and therefore deserve their own little blurbs. I eat a serving of each of these foods almost every day, and I consider them to be indispensable.

Avocados

Mentioning avocados almost seems cliché because they're so emblematic of both vegan and ketogenic diets. However, there's a reason for that. Avocados are loaded with vitamins and minerals, including significant amounts of potassium and the elusive B5. They're also absolutely delicious, especially when sprinkled with hemp seeds and nutritional yeast or Everything Bagel Blend (page 174).

In the recipes in this book, I use medium-sized Hass avocados, the edible portion of which weighs about 5 ounces (140 grams).

Frozen Spinach

Yes, frozen spinach. Spinach is a great source of vitamins A, C, and K, as well as manganese, iron, folate, potassium, and calcium. Frozen spinach is awesome because it's cost-effective, ready to go at a moment's notice with zero prep work, and super nutrient dense. I keep a few bags of spinach (as well as broccoli and cauliflower) in my freezer so that I can add more vegetables to smoothies and dinners with minimal effort.

Hulled Hemp Seeds (Hemp Hearts)

I can't say enough good things about hemp seeds. One serving (3 tablespoons/30 grams) contains 10 grams of protein and just 1 gram of net carbohydrates. These seeds also boast a pretty great omega-3 to omega-6 ratio and deliver significant quantities of magnesium, potassium, and zinc.

I use hemp seeds as the basis for a lot of sauces that normally would use higher-carb nuts like cashews, as well as add them to smoothies and sprinkle them on top of salads and yogurt.

Nutritional Yeast

Nutritional yeast imparts a "cheesy" flavor to foods. Just 2 tablespoons (10 grams) contains 8 grams of protein and a whole host of B vitamins, all for just 1 gram of net carbohydrates (although the carb counts may differ among brands!).

I tend to add nutritional yeast to creamy sauces and sprinkle it on top of roasted veggies, sliced avocados, and anything masquerading as spaghetti.

Sauerkraut

I *love* fermented foods, especially lacto-fermented* foods like sauerkraut. Not only is sauerkraut rich in sulfur compounds from the cabbage, but the process of fermentation effectively consumes the carbohydrates present in the cabbage. (Yay!)

Fermented foods have demonstrated a whole host of health benefits in studies,[67] from improved digestion and a reduction in inflammation[68] to improved mental health and moods.[69] Emerging research also suggests that certain strains of lactic bacteria even produce B vitamins as a by-product of the fermentation process.[70]

I tend to add sauerkraut to salads but also just put it on top of whatever else I'm eating.

---

*Lacto- *here refers to the bacteria strain* Lactobacillus *and is in no way related to dairy!*

Vegan Keto Shopping List

There's a common misconception that keto is an overly restrictive diet with little variety, and I would like to dispel that myth right now. As you can see on these two pages, ketogenic diets can include a kaleidoscope of veggies, nuts, seeds, and even beans and fruits.

 Fats

NUTS:

Almonds Ⓟ

Brazil nuts

Cashews Ⓖ

Hazelnuts *(also called filberts)*

Macadamia nuts

Peanuts *(I know, they're technically legumes…)*

Pecans

Pine nuts Ⓖ

Pistachios Ⓖ

Walnuts

SEEDS:

Chia seeds

Flax seeds

Hemp seeds Ⓟ

Pepitas (pumpkin seeds) Ⓟ

Sacha inchi seeds Ⓟ

Sunflower seeds Ⓟ

OTHER WHOLE-FOOD FAT SOURCES:

Avocados

Coconut

Olives

NUT & SEED BUTTERS*:

Almond butter Ⓟ

Coconut butter *(coconut manna)*

Hazelnut butter

Macadamia nut butter

Peanut butter Ⓟ

Pecan butter

Sunflower seed butter

Tahini

Walnut butter

*Be sure to look for unsweetened nut and seed butters!

HEALTHY OILS:

Almond oil

Avocado oil

Cacao butter *(great for body care and desserts!)*

Coconut oil

Extra-virgin olive oil

Flaxseed oil *(store in the fridge; not for cooking)*

Hazelnut oil

Macadamia nut oil

MCT oil *(for adding to smoothies, coffee, etc.)*

Walnut oil

 Produce

LOW-CARB VEGETABLES:

Artichoke hearts

Arugula

Asparagus

Beets Ⓖ

Bell peppers *(the green ones are the lowest in carbs)*

Bok choy

Broccoli

Broccoli rabe/raab/ rapini

Brussels sprouts Ⓖ

Cabbage

Carrots Ⓖ

Cauliflower

Celeriac *(also called celery root)* Ⓖ

Celery

Chard

Collards

Cucumbers

Daikon radish

Dandelion greens

Eggplant

Endive *(also called escarole)*

Fennel

Fiddleheads *(available for a short time in spring)*

Garlic

Jicama Ⓖ

Kale Ⓖ

Kohlrabi

Lettuce *(all types)*

Microgreens

Mushrooms

Mustard greens

Okra

Onions Ⓖ

Parsnips Ⓖ

Radishes

Rhubarb

Rutabaga Ⓖ

Shallots

Spinach

Sprouts *(all kinds)*

Squash—summer type *(crookneck, pattypan, zephyr)*

Squash—winter type *(butternut, pumpkin, spaghetti)* Ⓖ

Swiss chard

Turnips

Zucchini

LOW-CARB FRUITS:

Avocados

Blueberries Ⓖ

Coconut

Cranberries *(fresh or frozen, not dried)*

Lemons

Limes

Olives

Raspberries

Strawberries

Tomatoes

Watermelon Ⓖ

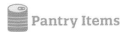 Pantry Items

Almond flour

Artichoke hearts

Baking powder

Baking soda

Cocoa or cacao powder

Coconut flour

Coconut milk *(canned full-fat)*

Dark chocolate *(85 percent cacao and up is usually super low in sugar, but be sure to check labels!)*

Flavorings and extracts *(check for added sugars)*

Hearts of palm

Jackfruit *(green, canned in brine, not syrup)*

Kelp flakes

Kelp noodles

Lupini beans *(jarred in brine)* ⓟ

Nori sheets

Nutritional yeast ⓟ

Psyllium husks *(whole husks tend to work better than powder for baking)*

Seasonings and spices *(check for added sugars or starch!)*

Seaweed snacks

Vanilla extract *(check for added sugars!)*

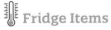 Fridge Items

Chili paste or hot sauce

Dairy-free cheese substitutes ⓒ

Dairy-free yogurt ⓒ *(unsweetened)*

Edamame ⓟ

Mustard

Pickles *(dill or other sugar-free types)*

Sauerkraut or vegan kimchi

Seitan ⓒ ⓟ *(if you can tolerate gluten)*

Shirataki noodles

Tamari or coconut aminos

Tempeh ⓟ

Tofu ⓟ

Tomato sauce *(check for added sugars!)*

Vinegars—apple cider, balsamic, rice wine, white wine

Wasabi paste *(check for hidden sugars or starch!)*

 Smoothie Add-Ins

Amla powder ⓒ

Beetroot powder ⓒ

Chlorella

Moringa

Mushroom extracts *(especially reishi, lion's mane, turkey tail, chaga, and cordyceps)*

Spirulina

Turmeric powder

❄ Freezer Items

Frozen berries

Frozen vegetables *(anything from the Low-Carb Vegetables list, opposite)*

Mock meats:

- Beyond Meat products
- Some Gardein products *(see Note below)*
- Some Quorn products *(see Note below)*

Riced cauliflower

Halo Top Dairy-Free Dessert ⓒ

Wink Frozen Dessert

Note: Some Gardein and Quorn products are both vegan and low-carb, but those that are breaded or come with a sauce tend to contain a whole day's worth of carbohydrates in one serving! Additionally, many Quorn products contain egg.

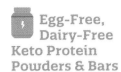 Egg-Free, Dairy-Free Keto Protein Powders & Bars

Garden of Life RAW

Julian Bakery Pegan Bars

Nugo Slim Vegan Bars ⓒ

Plain hemp protein powder

Plain pea protein powder

Plain soy protein powder

Raw Revolution Glo Bars ⓒ

Sun Warrior Classic Plus

Sun Warrior Warrior Blend

Vega Clean Protein

Vega Sport Protein

Shopping list notes:

- *Foods marked with a ⓒ are a little higher in carbs and should be consumed sparingly.*
- *Foods marked with a ⓟ are good sources of protein.*
- *It's always good to read the labels on the foods you buy, especially on processed foods like nondairy milk, cheese, yogurt, and mock meats.*
- *If a food is not included in this list, it doesn't mean that it can't be consumed on keto—just be sure to check the carb count!*
- *You can find more details about some of the foods in this list under "Special Ingredients" on pages 52 to 55.*

Tools & Equipment

While cooking food on a vegan keto diet doesn't necessarily require special tools, there are a few things that can help simplify your life in the kitchen. I assume that you already have basic kitchen tools like a cutting board, measuring spoons, and various pots and pans; this list just suggests some tools that will make vegan keto cooking a bit easier.

Sharp Knife

If you plan on doing a lot of cooking, make sure you have a sharp knife. Having an actual chef's knife can cut your food prep time in half. Using a sharp knife is safer than using a dull one, too!

Mandoline Slicer

If I were to recommend just one kitchen tool, it would be a mandoline slicer with a few different blades. For those who are unfamiliar with this tool, a mandoline enables you to quickly and uniformly slice and julienne vegetables. Some models even have grating and "french fry cut" settings. They are pretty inexpensive (mine cost less than $10) and definitely save you time in the kitchen.

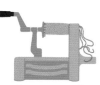

Vegetable Spiral Slicer

If you find yourself making veggie noodles with any frequency, a spiral slicer is a huge time-saver. These run the gamut from large countertop slicers that you turn with a hand crank to small handheld ones that are very reasonably priced and can fit in a drawer. I own a small one that doesn't take much effort to clean and comes in handy when I want to make Zucchini Alfredo (page 150).

Kitchen Scale

If you've been thinking about investing in a kitchen scale, I definitely recommend going for it. Not only will weighing your food give you more accurate portion sizes, but you'll have more success with baking as well. While the volume of an ingredient can change based on how it's measured, 100 grams of coconut flour will always weigh 100 grams. I prefer to weigh out ingredients like flour, protein powder, cocoa powder, psyllium husks, and ground nuts and seeds that tend to clump together or settle, making precise volumetric measuring difficult.

Blender

About five years ago, I bought myself a high-powered blender during a 40 percent off sale (how could I not?), and it has been truly life-changing. I use it for making pretty much everything, from nut butters to soups to sauces to ice cream. It's rare that a day goes by when I don't fire up the ol' gal to do some serious blending.

If a high-powered blender isn't in the cards for you, a regular blender is still an incredibly helpful tool to have. While most of the recipes in this book that involve blending can be made with a normal countertop blender, the Lupini Hummus (page 93) and the Keto Pot Pie (page 138) really do require a high-powered blender to become totally smooth.

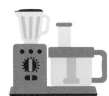

Food Processor

If you're not ready to make the leap and purchase a high-powered blender, then I definitely recommend buying a food processor that holds at least 2 cups (about 500 ml). Making nut flours and sauces and finely chopping anything is so much easier with a food processor.

Garlic Press

I'm normally pretty opposed to cluttering up my kitchen with "unitaskers." Aside from crushing garlic, there's not much that a garlic press can do. However, I really don't love smashing and finely chopping cloves of garlic, so for me, the utility of a garlic press is well worth the drawer space it takes up.

A good grater can take the place of a garlic press. It takes a little longer to use but less time to clean.

Grater

A fine grater (like a Microplane) is so helpful for grating ginger and zesting citrus fruits and can even replace a garlic press.

Citrus Juicer

This is another unitasker, but after fishing countless lemon seeds out of dressings, sauces, and batters, I caved and bought one for a whole $4. I'm not talking about a giant citrus press that sits on your counter, but rather a little glass or plastic device that sits atop a cup or bowl and catches the seeds when you squeeze the juice from citrus fruits. If you use a lot of lemon juice, this gadget is worth having for sure.

Coffee or Spice Grinder

Even if you don't grind your own coffee, you will find plenty of uses for a coffee or spice grinder. It's great for grinding flax seeds, spices that are purchased whole (like cardamom), and granulated sweeteners for recipes in which the powdered form is preferred.

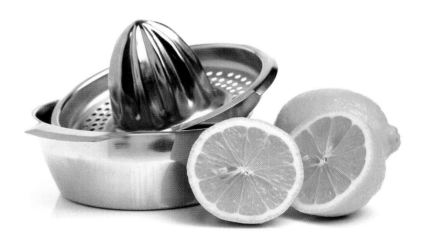

Special Ingredients

For the recipes in this book, I wanted to use ingredients that are widely available. It's no fun getting ready to make a recipe and then realizing that one of the key ingredients can be purchased only at a health food store or online. So I bought all the ingredients I used to make these recipes at the grocery store down the street from me—not a health food store, not a specialty vegan website, but a regular grocery store.

Some of the ingredients used in these recipes are of a specific variety, and others aren't particularly common (especially if you are new to vegan or ketogenic eating or both), so I thought it would be worth giving you some more information about them.

Nut & Seed Butters

The almond and peanut butters that I use are creamy, unsweetened, salted, and usually labeled "natural." The best options contain just nuts and salt, with no added oils or sweeteners. A little stirring is often necessary to redistribute the oil evenly throughout the butter.

I use a lot of nut and seed butters, so I keep them at room temperature so that they're ready for use in recipes. If you prefer to store your nut and seed butters in the fridge, be sure to measure out the necessary amount for your recipe and let it reach room temperature before using it.

Coconut Milk

You will see two different types of coconut milk used in these recipes: full-fat canned coconut milk and unsweetened coconut milk. The difference is important for making the recipes successfully and for tracking your macros accurately!

Full-fat canned coconut milk is thick and rich and (obviously) found in cans. Most supermarkets stock this product in two places—with the other nondairy milks that are packaged in shelf-stable containers and with the Thai specialty foods. Be sure to buy the full-fat version instead of light or "lite" canned coconut milk, as the latter contains less fat and more liquid and doesn't work the same way in many recipes.

Unsweetened coconut milk is thinner and functions more like almond milk, soy milk, and other nondairy milks that you see in cartons and boxes. Typically, grocery stores carry unsweetened coconut milk in two locations—refrigerated in the dairy case and in shelf-stable packaging, often in the cereal aisle. There are many brands available, and some brands even offer vanilla and chocolate flavors.

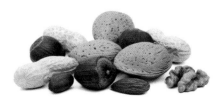

Coconut Oil
With very few exceptions, I use unrefined, cold-pressed coconut oil for cooking and baking. This oil, which comes from the first pressing of the fruit, contains more nutrients and phytochemicals than refined coconut oil. Unrefined coconut oil does have a bit of a coconutty taste, though. So, if you really don't want the taste of coconut in your food, then you may want to opt for the refined type. Whether or not the oil is refined doesn't impact its texture or any aspect of the finished product other than nutrient content and taste.

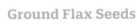
Crushed Garlic
A lot of the recipes in this book call for crushed garlic. I crush garlic using a garlic press or a Microplane grater, but you can achieve the same effect with a knife and cutting board: Mince the garlic, sprinkle with a little salt (to provide an abrasion), then use the side of the blade to firmly press the minced garlic across the cutting board. Scrape the garlic into a mound, then repeat the mincing and pressing actions until you have a paste.

Ground Flax Seeds
While you can buy flax seeds preground, I prefer to buy whole flax seeds and grind them as needed for each recipe. This keeps the seeds fresh longer.

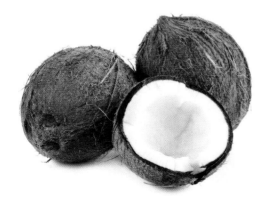

Granulated Sweetener
Many recipes in this book call for granulated sweetener. I look for brands that are made with erythritol as the base, as this sugar alcohol closely mimics sugar in cooking and baking. There are many brands out there, but the ones I have tried with success are Lakanto, Swerve, and Sukrin. You'll notice that all of these sweeteners are erythritol blends and not pure erythritol.

If you are converting a sugar-based recipe to make it keto-friendly, I've found that using the same amount of granulated sweetener is a little overpowering. I usually use between one-third and one-half the amount of sweetener called for in the non-keto recipe.

Sometimes a recipe works better when you use a powdered sweetener instead of a granulated one. Frostings are a good example. In these cases, I make my own powdered sweetener by grinding some granulated sweetener in a coffee or spice grinder. Just be sure to clean out the grinder afterward unless you like your coffee to be overwhelmingly sweet! Trust me here.

Xylitol-based sweeteners also can work well in recipes, but they tend to be a little harsher on people's digestive systems. Additionally, xylitol is highly toxic to pets, so be sure to keep any baked goods containing xylitol away from your animal friends!

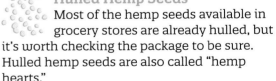
Hulled Hemp Seeds
Most of the hemp seeds available in grocery stores are already hulled, but it's worth checking the package to be sure. Hulled hemp seeds are also called "hemp hearts."

Jackfruit

Jackfruit is one of those fun foods that emulates a meaty texture pretty effectively. It's usually used in place of chicken or pulled pork in vegan versions of traditional recipes. For example, you'll find it in my Keto Pot Pie (page 138) and my Buffalo Jackfruit Tacos (page 151).

As the name implies, jackfruit is a fruit. It grows in lowland tropical climates and is a common ingredient in South Asian and Southeast Asian cooking. While the mature fruit is high in carbs and sugar, young, green jackfruit is keto-friendly. Make sure that you are buying this young variety and that it is packed in brine. Mature jackfruit is often packed in sugar syrup.

You can find canned green jackfruit in the imported foods aisle at most grocery stores, including chains like Trader Joe's. Some brands are even starting to make seasoned packaged jackfruit that's ready to add to meals. Just be sure to check the carb count on the back of the package!

Liquid Stevia

In addition to erythritol-based granulated sweeteners, I sometimes use liquid stevia in recipes. There are plenty of brands out there; I usually end up buying the private-label ones from Whole Foods Market or Trader Joe's.

Some people prefer to use powdered stevia because it tends to contain fewer ingredients (and is often just pure extract), but I prefer the liquid form because it is less likely to clump and create a wholly unpleasant-tasting experience. I also like the liquid form because you can add just a few drops at a time and dial in the sweetness. Too much stevia can make foods taste bitter, so it's best to start with less than you think you'll need and add a few drops at a time.

Lupini Beans

Also called lupins, these beans have been found in ancient Egyptian tombs and are now most frequently consumed in the Mediterranean and Latin America. Lupins are pretty low in carbs, especially for beans, and contain a significant amount of lysine.

If not properly soaked in brine for several days, these beans are strongly bitter. For this reason, I tend to buy them already brined. You can find brined lupini beans in most grocery stores with the Latin American or Italian foods, packaged in jars.

A quick note: There is some cross-reactivity between lupini beans and peanuts, so those with peanut allergies may want to avoid them!

Nondairy Milks

In addition to coconut milk, there are plenty of other milk substitutes on the market (with more coming out all the time!). In the recipes in this book, these other nondairy milks can be used interchangeably. So, if you really don't like almond milk, feel free to use something else.

Often, grocery stores stock nondairy milks in two sections—the refrigerated dairy section and in shelf-stable packaging near the breakfast cereals. Be sure to buy the unsweetened kind, as the sweetened versions often contain quite a bit of sugar.

I really like and often use pea milk because it provides far more protein per cup than most other nondairy milks. The brand I usually buy is Ripple, and it's found in the refrigerated dairy section.

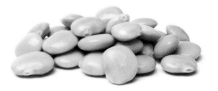

Nut & Seed Flours

Nut and seed flours are a key ingredient in many keto baked goods. I like to make my own flours to save money. Making your own nut or seed flour is as simple as placing the nuts or seeds in a food processor or high-powered blender and processing them until they have the texture of sand. For nuts with skins, like almonds or hazelnuts, using blanched nuts will give your flour a nicer appearance and a finer texture.

Many nut flours can be used interchangeably. For example, almond flour can be replaced by hazelnut flour, cashew flour, or macadamia nut flour in baked goods. If you are avoiding nuts, you can use ground seeds (like sunflower seeds or pepitas/pumpkin seeds) instead.

Store your homemade nut and seed flours in a sealed container in the refrigerator for up to two weeks. For more on how I make and store nut and seed flours, check out page 176.

Olive Oil

I buy cold-pressed extra-virgin olive oil for use in cooking. This is the oil that comes from the first pressing of the olives and contains the most nutrients and phytochemicals.

Look for olive oil that is packaged in dark-colored bottles, and be sure to store it in a cool, dry place at a constant temperature to prevent oxidation.

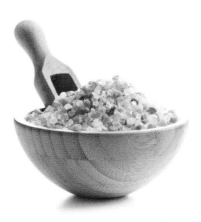

Pea Protein & Other Protein Powders

I use pea protein in a few recipes in this book. I like pea protein because it contains a solid amount of lysine (refer to page 17 for more on lysine) and doesn't tend to present an issue allergen-wise, like soy and rice proteins do.

If you are unable to consume pea protein, you can substitute another vegan protein powder of your choosing. For baked goods, hemp seed protein works well as a substitute for pea protein. For smoothies and other treats, you can use any vegan protein powder you like. There are many different brands of vegan protein powders and blends that are low in carbohydrates—just be sure to check the labels!

You can find protein powders at health food stores and many online retailers, as well as your regular grocery store.

Salt

Because people who follow a ketogenic diet tend to need more minerals than other people, I recommend using a less-refined salt like Celtic sea salt or pink Himalayan salt that contains trace minerals. I typically use a finely ground salt unless otherwise noted in a recipe.

Tamari

Tamari is basically gluten-free soy sauce. I like to buy the low-sodium variety, which contains about one-third less sodium than regular tamari. If you are unable to consume soy, coconut aminos can be used as a substitute for tamari in any recipe in this book.

Tempeh

Tempeh is made from fermented soybeans and has a much firmer texture than tofu. You can find many different varieties in most grocery stores, often in the produce section alongside the tofu. Tempeh is sometimes made with other ingredients as well, from flax seeds to quinoa and grains, so be sure to check the nutrition label for the carb count.

Using the Recipes in This Book

Like most of you, I'm not a professional chef. So all of the recipes in this book are meant for regular people with regular kitchens. I also don't love doing dishes (and don't have a dishwasher), so I try not to use too many unnecessary bowls or pans in meal prep.

Because I know that a lot of you don't have hours every day to spend in the kitchen, I have provided plenty of quick and easy recipes that can be made in less than fifteen minutes. Of course, there are also recipes that do involve more steps and require some extra pans, because I really love cooking and experimenting in the kitchen, and I know a lot of you do, too.

You'll notice some icons at the tops of the recipes. These icons indicate that the recipe is free of certain allergens:

 • **Coconut-free**

 • **Nut-free**

 • **Peanut-free**

 • **Soy-free**

Because every recipe in this book is dairy-free, egg-free, gluten-free, and wheat-free, there are no icons for these foods.

I have also provided nutrition information for each recipe. These calculations take only the base recipe into account and exclude optional ingredients. I gathered the ingredient information from the United States Department of Agriculture Food Composition Database and a few select food labels when no database entry was available. While I strove to be as accurate as possible, nutrition information can vary among varieties of foods as well as brands, so your calculations may vary slightly.

Storage and reheating instructions are also provided to make life that much easier.

Measuring Ingredients

All recipes in this book include both imperial volumetric measurements and their metric weight or volume equivalents for quantities of 2 tablespoons or greater.

While I often use a kitchen scale to measure ingredients, when I'm using volumetric measurements like cups and tablespoons, I scoop the ingredient out of the container and then scrape off the excess with the back of a knife. So, unless specifically stated, measurements are not "rounded" or heaping cups or tablespoons.

Yes, I already mentioned a kitchen scale in the tools section, but I think it's an important enough tool to list twice. Baking without butter, eggs, dairy milk, sugar, or traditional flour can be really tricky, so weighing your ingredients helps eliminate at least one variable. The volume of an ingredient can vary depending on how you measure it, and with ingredients like coconut flour and psyllium husks, even a slight variance can make a big difference in the final dish. A kitchen scale isn't too expensive and really helps ensure that your recipes turn out consistently.

Making Substitutions

I know that many of you are nut-free or soy-free or have allergies or sensitivities that go beyond eggs, dairy, and gluten (which aren't used in these recipes). The good news is that most substitutions are fairly simple:

 Note:

The allergen icons used in the recipes are based on the first ingredient choice listed. In many cases, you can use the second ingredient listed to make the recipe coconut-free, nut-free, peanut-free, or soy-free to meet your dietary needs. For example, a recipe that calls for tamari or coconut aminos will be marked with the coconut-free icon. If you do not eat soy but are okay with coconut, simply use coconut aminos instead.

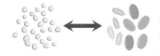 Ground flax seeds and ground chia seeds can be used interchangeably.

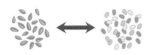 Hemp seeds can easily be replaced by sunflower seeds or pepitas (pumpkin seeds) in many recipes.

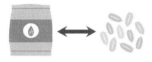 Nuts can often be replaced with sunflower seeds (in the case of "walnut meat" and almond flour).

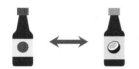 Tamari can be replaced with coconut aminos.

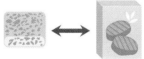 Tempeh and tofu can be replaced by soy-free mock meats.

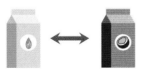 Almond milk can be replaced with coconut milk or another nut-free nondairy milk.

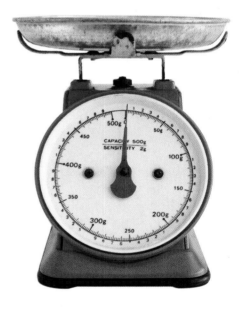

DO I HAVE TO MAKE EVERYTHING FROM SCRATCH?

In this book, you'll notice recipes for dressings, spreads, and condiments that can also be store-bought. While the homemade versions are typically much more nutrient dense, there's nothing wrong with using a premade variety to save time! Just be sure to check the label for hidden carbs.

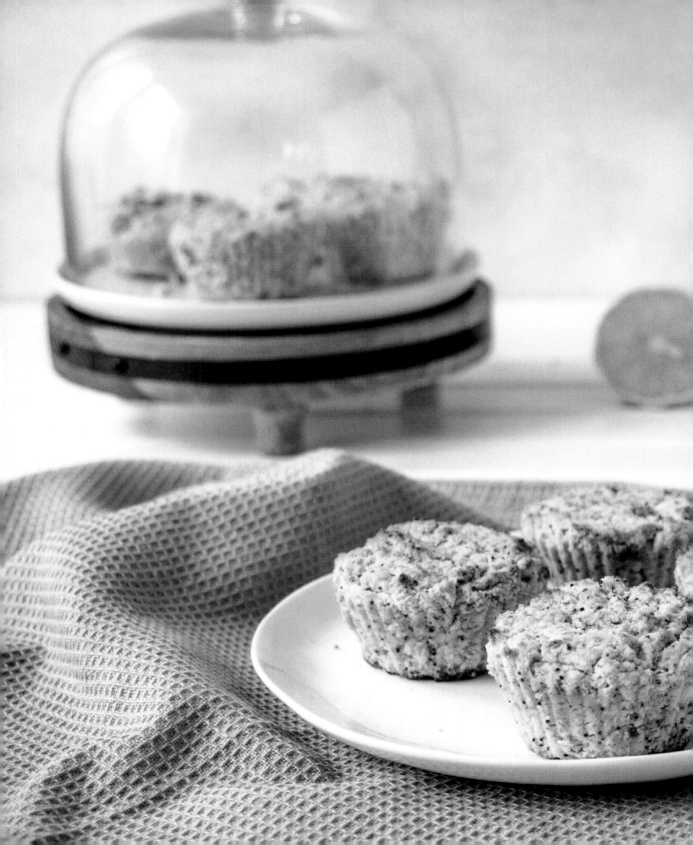

Breakfast

Coconut Flour Waffles

Waffles are most definitely my desert island food. I could eat them night and day. These waffles make me extra happy because they are both gluten-free and nut-free. While they're really tasty fresh off the waffle iron, they also toast up nicely should you want to reheat leftovers the next day.

YIELD: 4 mini waffles, 2 regular waffles, or 1 Belgian waffle (2 servings)
PREP TIME: 10 minutes   COOK TIME: 5 to 20 minutes

2 tablespoons (28g) coconut oil, softened, plus extra for the waffle iron

1 tablespoon granulated sweetener

¼ cup (28g) coconut flour

1 tablespoon psyllium husks

½ teaspoon baking powder

Pinch of salt

½ cup (120 ml) unsweetened coconut milk or other nondairy milk of choice

1 teaspoon vanilla extract

TOPPING SUGGESTIONS:

Coconut cream (see Note, page 162)

Fresh raspberries, strawberries, or blackberries

Ground cinnamon or cocoa powder

Keto Buttery Spread (page 187) or vegan butter substitute of choice

- Preheat a waffle iron according to the manufacturer's instructions. Be sure to grease the waffle iron with coconut oil so that the waffles don't stick!

- In a small mixing bowl, fork-whisk the coconut oil and sweetener until smooth and fluffy.

- In another small bowl, whisk together the coconut flour, psyllium husks, baking powder, and salt. Add the dry ingredients to the coconut oil and sweetener and use the fork to mash until the mixture has the texture of wet sand.

- Pour in the coconut milk and vanilla extract and stir until any large lumps disappear. Let sit for 3 to 5 minutes, until the milk is completely absorbed, then stir again to remove any remaining lumps. The mixture won't be totally smooth, as the coconut flour is somewhat textured, and it will be quite thick, more like a dough than a batter.

- Divide the dough into 2 equal portions to make 2 regular-size waffles or into 4 equal portions to make 4 mini waffles. If using a Belgian waffle maker, leave the dough in one piece to make a single large waffle.

- Roll the portion of dough into a ball before placing it in the center of the waffle iron. Cook for about 5 minutes, until golden brown.

- Carefully remove the waffle from the waffle iron. I like to (carefully) shimmy a chopstick under the waffle to loosen it a little, then free it using 2 forks for support.

- Repeat with any remaining dough.

- Top as desired and serve.

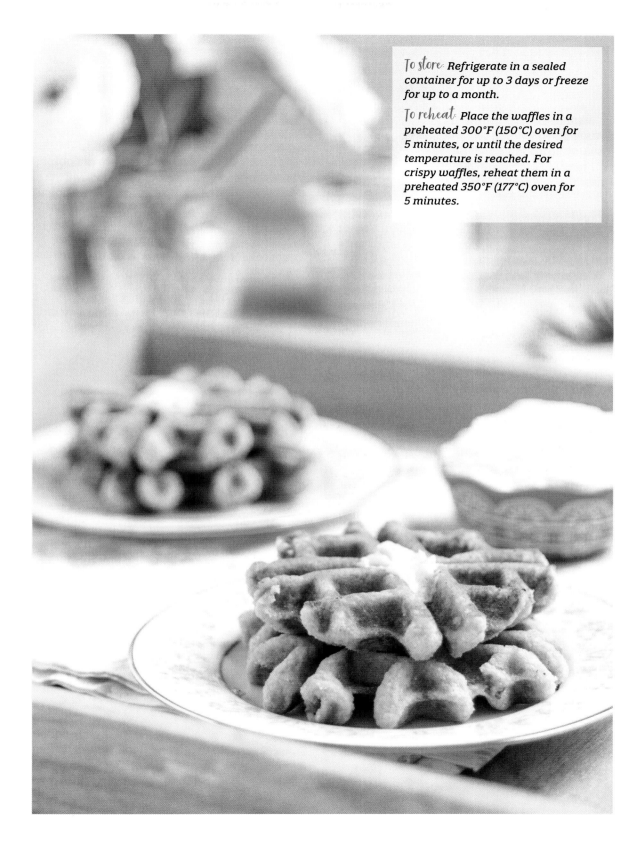

To store: Refrigerate in a sealed container for up to 3 days or freeze for up to a month.

To reheat: Place the waffles in a preheated 300°F (150°C) oven for 5 minutes, or until the desired temperature is reached. For crispy waffles, reheat them in a preheated 350°F (177°C) oven for 5 minutes.

Spinach & Olive Mini Quiche Cups

While these mini crustless quiches are great for breakfast, there's no reason they can't be enjoyed for lunch or dinner! Tofu works well here to give them an egglike texture while also bringing some protein to the table. On weekends when I have a little more time to make breakfast, I whip these up along with some Sausage-Style Breakfast Patties (page 64) and enjoy them with sliced avocado.

I used Kalamata olives for this recipe, but it can be fun to try out other types in their place. The antipasto bars at many supermarkets usually have several different types of olives, often in interesting marinades. Just by changing the olives, you can really change up the flavor profile of this dish.

YIELD: 8 mini quiches (2 per serving) PREP TIME: 10 minutes, plus at least 10 minutes to cool COOK TIME: 45 minutes

1 (14-ounce/397-g) block extra-firm tofu

¼ cup plus 2 tablespoons (30g) nutritional yeast

2 tablespoons (30 ml) extra-virgin olive oil, plus extra for the pan

2 tablespoons (30 ml) water

1 teaspoon garlic powder

½ teaspoon onion powder

¼ teaspoon ground black pepper

½ teaspoon salt

1 teaspoon baking powder

4 ounces (112g) pitted Kalamata olives, chopped

3 lightly packed cups (90g) chopped fresh spinach, or ½ cup (90g) thawed frozen spinach

Sliced scallions (green parts only), for garnish (optional)

- Preheat the oven to 350°F (177°C) and grease 8 wells of a standard-size muffin pan with olive oil.

- In a food processor or blender, process the tofu with the nutritional yeast, olive oil, water, spices, salt, and baking powder until the mixture has a smooth hummuslike consistency.

- Transfer the tofu mixture to a medium-sized mixing bowl and stir in the olives and spinach, making sure to break up any large clumps of spinach so that everything is evenly distributed.

- Fill the muffin cups about three-quarters of the way full. Bake for 45 minutes, until the edges of the quiches are slightly golden and a thin crust forms over the top.

- Remove from the oven and let cool in the pan for at least 10 minutes to give the quiches time to set up. Once cool, they should slide out of the pan easily. (*Note:* The easiest way to remove them is to hold a cooling rack flush to the top of the muffin pan and carefully invert it. When you lift the pan, the quiches should be on the cooling rack.)

- Serve warm or at room temperature. Garnish with sliced scallions, if desired.

To store: Refrigerate in a sealed container for up to 3 days or freeze for up to a month.

To reheat: While the leftovers are delicious cold, these mini quiches can be warmed in a preheated 300°F (150°C) oven for 10 minutes, or until the desired temperature is reached.

NUTRITION INFORMATION: **277** calories | **19.7g** fat | **17.3g** protein | **10.1g** total carbs | **3.6g** net carbs

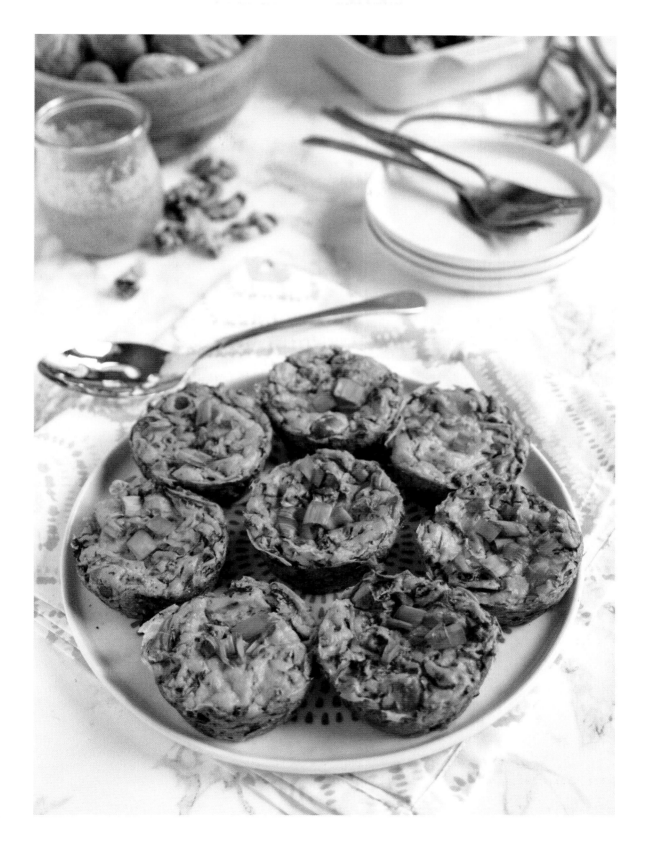

Sausage-Style Breakfast Patties

I'm a huge fan of savory breakfast and brunch options. Muffins, waffles, and smoothies are great, but sometimes you want something a little less sweet. My favorite way to eat these sausage-style patties is sandwiched in a Tahini Bagel (page 80) with some arugula and sauerkraut as a vegan keto breakfast sandwich.

YIELD: 8 patties (2 per serving)   PREP TIME: 10 minutes (not including time to make spice blend)   COOK TIME: 25 minutes

1 cup (120g) raw walnuts, chopped

½ cup (56g) ground flax seeds

½ cup (120 ml) vegetable broth

2 teaspoons Sausage Spice Blend (page 172)

- Preheat the oven to 350°F (177°C) and line a rimmed baking sheet with parchment paper.

- In a small mixing bowl, stir together all the ingredients until thoroughly combined. Let sit for about 5 minutes, until a thick, sticky dough forms.

- Divide the dough into 8 equal portions, then form each portion into a 3-inch (8-cm) round patty.

- Place the patties on the lined baking sheet and bake for 25 minutes, until firm to the touch. Serve warm.

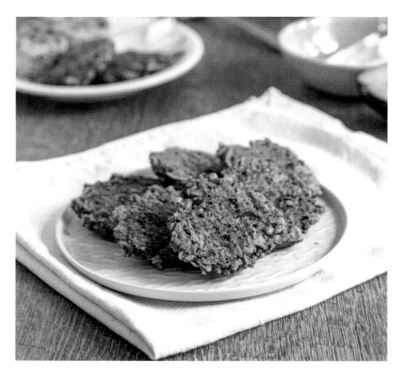

To store Refrigerate in a sealed container for up to 3 days or freeze for up to a month.

To reheat Place the patties in a preheated 300°F (150°C) oven for 10 minutes, or until the desired temperature is reached.

NUTRITION INFORMATION: **275** calories | **25.5g** fat | **7.3g** protein | **9.2g** total carbs | **3.2g** net carbs

High-Protein "Noatmeal"

This hearty bowl is my go-to meal when I have a big day ahead of me. It is high in fat and protein and fills me up for quite a while. When I've got an especially busy week ahead, I'll prep several jars with just the dry ingredients and then add the liquid ingredients as needed to make Overnight "Noats" throughout the week (see the Variation below). I like to top mine with pepitas, coconut yogurt, and sometimes even a few berries.

YIELD: 1 serving   PREP TIME: 2 minutes   COOK TIME: 5 minutes

¾ cup (180 ml) unsweetened coconut milk or other nondairy milk of choice

¼ cup (40g) hulled hemp seeds

2 tablespoons (14g) ground flax seeds

2 tablespoons (14g) pea protein powder or other vegan protein powder of choice

¼ teaspoon ground cinnamon, plus extra for sprinkling

½ teaspoon vanilla extract

⅛ teaspoon liquid stevia

TOPPING SUGGESTIONS:

Fresh berries

Raw or roasted pepitas (pumpkin seeds)

Coconut Yogurt (page 68)

Put all the ingredients except the vanilla extract and stevia in a small saucepan and stir to combine. Heat gently over medium heat just until the milk is bubbling around the edges of the pan, then remove from the heat. Let the mixture sit for about a minute to thicken and cool. Stir in the vanilla and stevia, then pour into a serving bowl and sprinkle with a little cinnamon. Top with fresh berries, pepitas, and/or yogurt, if desired.

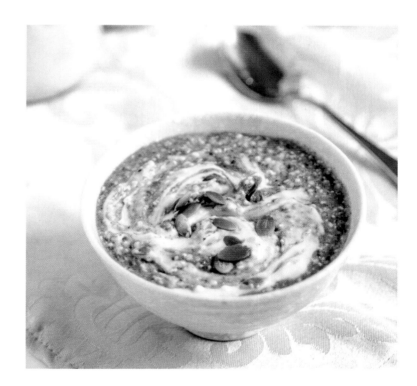

Variation OVERNIGHT "NOATS."
Stir all the ingredients together in a pint jar (475 ml) and refrigerate overnight. Enjoy the "noats" chilled, straight from the fridge, the next morning.

NUTRITION INFORMATION: **385** calories | **26.9g** fat | **27.4g** protein | **9.1g** total carbs | **3.1g** net carbs

Nut-Free Chocolate Granola

Growing up in the nineties instilled in me a strong desire for chocolatey breakfast foods. Chocolate peanut butter puffed cereal, chocolate meal replacement shakes, and chocolate chip mini muffins made frequent appearances in my breakfast lineup. I like to think that this chocolate granola is a more refined version of those hyper-sugary treats, with omega-3 fatty acids, protein, and fiber to boot! I usually add this to a bowl of Coconut Yogurt (page 68) or eat it like cereal with whatever nondairy milk I have on hand.

  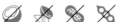

YIELD: 4 cups (200g) (about ¾ cup/40g per serving)
PREP TIME: 5 minutes   COOK TIME: 20 minutes

2 tablespoons (24g) granulated sweetener

1 rounded tablespoon cocoa powder

1 tablespoon water

1 tablespoon tahini, room temperature

Pinch of salt

½ cup (80g) hulled hemp seeds

½ cup (60g) raw pepitas (pumpkin seeds)

¼ cup (40g) sesame seeds

- Preheat the oven to 300°F (150°C) and line a rimmed baking sheet with parchment paper.

- In a medium-sized mixing bowl, whisk together the sweetener, cocoa powder, water, tahini, and salt until fully blended.

- Add all the seeds to the bowl and mix with a rubber spatula until the seeds are completely coated in the chocolate mixture and the ingredients come together to form a slightly crumbly dough.

- Spread the mixture on the lined baking sheet in an even layer, making sure to keep some clusters intact.

- Bake for 20 minutes, until the clusters are firm to the touch and no longer sticky.

- Let cool completely before transferring to an airtight container.

To store **Keep in an airtight container in a dry place for up to 5 days.**

NUTRITION INFORMATION: **225** calories | **20.2g** fat | **10.8g** protein | **9.4g** total carbs | **2g** net carbs

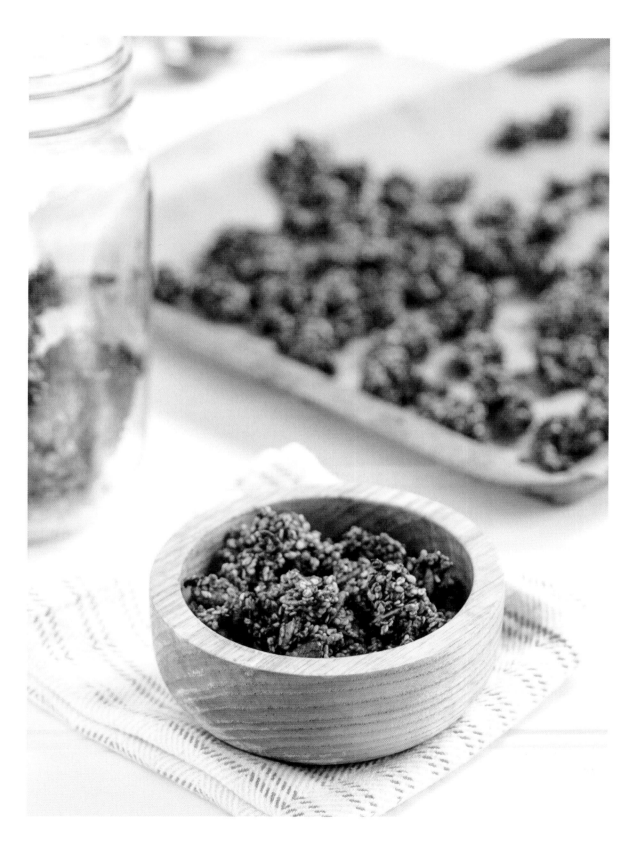

Coconut Yogurt

This homemade yogurt tastes better than any I've found at the store and is so easy to make! You don't even need a yogurt maker. While you can use any brand of canned coconut milk you like, I've had the greatest success with those brands that contain guar gum.

YIELD: 1⅔ cups (400 ml) (heaping ½ cup/120 ml per serving)
PREP TIME: 5 minutes, plus 24 to 48 hours to ferment

1 (13.5-ounce/400-ml) can full-fat coconut milk

1 or more probiotic capsules (see Notes)

- Pour the coconut milk and contents of the probiotic capsule(s) into a blender or food processor. Process until smooth and well combined, 10 to 20 seconds, depending on how solid the coconut milk was.

- Pour the mixture into a clean, dry pint jar (475 ml), cover the top with cheesecloth, and secure it with a rubber band.

- Place the jar in a relatively warm place (at least 70°F/21°C) out of direct sunlight for 24 to 48 hours, depending on the desired consistency and flavor (see Notes). I usually check it at 24 hours, then every 4 to 6 hours after that.

- Once the fermentation is complete, seal the lid on the jar and place in the refrigerator. The yogurt will set up slightly more once chilled.

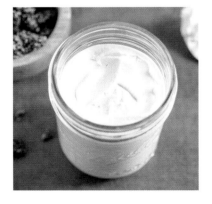

To store *Refrigerate for up to a week.*

Notes *The type of probiotic capsule used and the fermentation time will determine how thick and tangy the yogurt is. I used the contents of one probiotic capsule that provided 30 billion colony-forming units (CFUs). In 48 hours, I had a tangy yogurt with a thick and creamy texture similar to Greek yogurt.*

For an even thicker yogurt, increase the probiotic bacteria. While there isn't a perfect formula for achieving a certain consistency, if the temperature of the room remains consistent, doubling the number of CFUs to 60 billion should yield a thick coconut yogurt in half the time.

For a thinner, less tangy yogurt, use just 1 probiotic capsule (30 billion CFUs) and transfer the yogurt to the fridge after 24 hours.

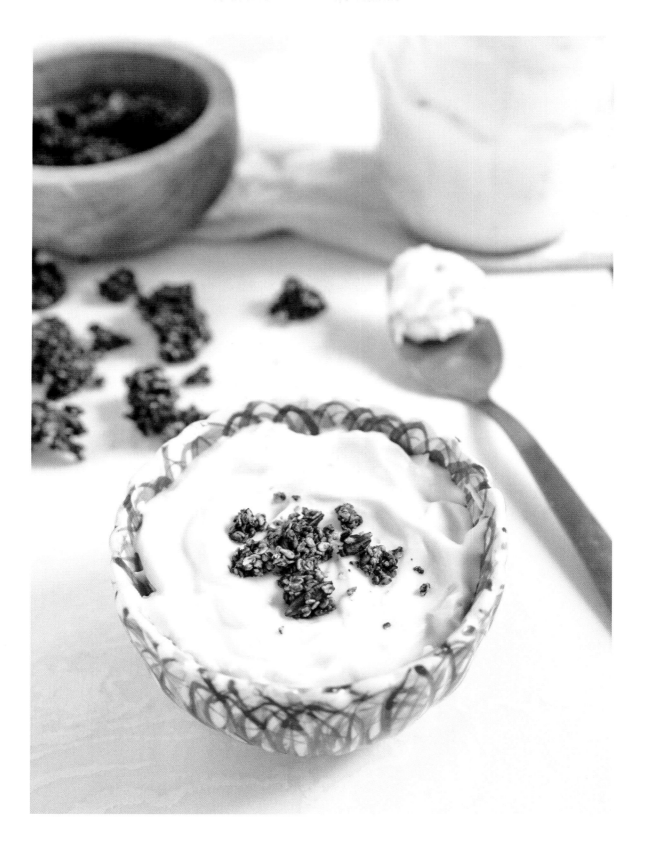

Lemon Poppy Seed Muffins

When I first went keto, the thing I missed most about eating a high-carb diet was baked goods. Baking is one of my absolute favorite activities. In college, I started a cupcake delivery service for the briefest of moments, and then later I worked in a bakery. Learning how to bake without gluten, eggs, dairy, and now sugar and grain flours has been an adventure, but the results are so worth the effort. These lemony muffins really brighten my day. I enjoy baking them on weekends and eating them topped with some Keto Buttery Spread (page 187), accompanied by a Coconut Matcha Latte (page 158).

YIELD: 5 muffins (1 per serving)
PREP TIME: 10 minutes   COOK TIME: 30 minutes

¾ cup (180 ml) coconut milk or other nondairy milk of choice

Grated zest and juice of 1 lemon

3 tablespoons (36g) granulated sweetener

2 tablespoons (30 ml) extra-virgin olive oil

1 teaspoon vanilla extract

½ cup (56g) ground flax seeds (see Tip)

½ cup (56g) coconut flour

1 teaspoon poppy seeds

1 teaspoon baking powder

⅛ teaspoon baking soda

Pinch of salt

- Preheat the oven to 375°F (190°C) and line 5 wells of a standard-size muffin pan with paper liners. Alternatively, use an unlined silicone muffin pan.

- In a small mixing bowl, whisk together the nondairy milk, lemon zest and juice, sweetener, olive oil, and vanilla extract.

- In a separate small bowl, use a fork to whisk together the remaining ingredients.

- Quickly stir the wet ingredients into the dry ingredients until no clumps remain and the mixture is thickened and aerated. Stop mixing to preserve this volume.

- Carefully scoop the batter into the lined wells of the muffin pan, filling them to the top, and bake for 30 minutes, until a knife comes out clean and the tops of the muffins are firm to the touch.

- Remove from the oven and let cool in the pan for at least 15 minutes so the muffins have time to set up.

- Once cool, the muffins should easily pop out of the pan. If you used a silicone muffin pan, run a knife around the inside of each well once the muffins have cooled to ensure easy removal.

To store **Keep in a sealed container at room temperature for up to 3 days or refrigerate for up to 5 days.**

Tip **Using golden flax seeds will give your baked goods a lighter appearance, more consistent with that of traditional baked goods.**

Variation LEMON BLUEBERRY MUFFINS. **Replace the poppy seeds with ¼ cup (40g) of fresh blueberries.**

NUTRITION INFORMATION: **169** calories | **12.5g** fat | **4.8g** protein | **17.1g** total carbs | **2.4g** net carbs

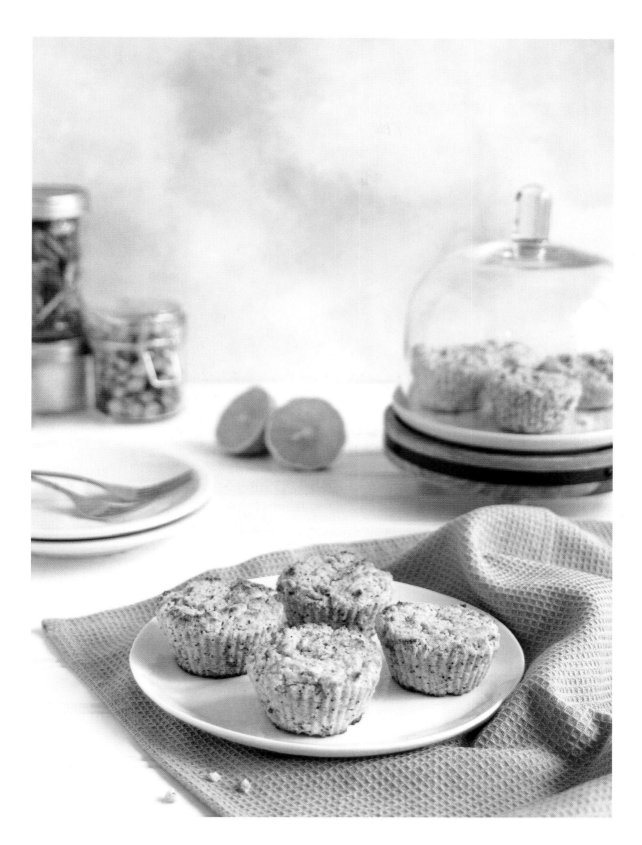

Pumpkin Bread

There's something so comforting about a warm slice of pumpkin bread, especially on a cool fall morning with a nice hot cup of coffee. I enjoy topping this bread with Keto Buttery Spread (page 187).

To make this bread soy-free, replace the soy flour with an equal measure of chickpea flour, fava bean flour, or lupin flour. Just be sure to account for the difference in carbohydrates!

YIELD: one 9 by 5-inch (23 by 12.75-cm) loaf (8 servings)
PREP TIME: 10 minutes   COOK TIME: 50 minutes

⅓ cup (80 ml) coconut milk or other nondairy milk of choice

¼ cup (48g) granulated sweetener

2 tablespoons (14g) ground flax seeds

1 teaspoon vanilla extract

¾ cup (170g) pumpkin puree

½ cup (112g) coconut oil, softened

¾ cup (84g) soy flour

¼ cup (28g) coconut flour

2 teaspoons ground cinnamon

½ teaspoon baking powder

¼ teaspoon baking soda

¼ teaspoon salt

To store *Keep covered at room temperature for up to 2 days, cover and refrigerate for up to 4 days, or slice and freeze for up to a month.*

To reheat *Reheat frozen slices in a preheated 350°F (177°C) oven for about 5 minutes, until warmed through, or for up to 10 minutes to toast them.*

Tip *Freeze the remaining half can of pumpkin puree for a future batch of this bread, or use it to make pumpkin spice lattes (page 159).*

- Preheat the oven to 350°F (177°C) and line a 9 by 5-inch (23 by 12.75-cm) loaf pan with parchment paper. Leave at least 2 inches (5 cm) of extra parchment on each long side of the pan for easier removal of the loaf.

- In a medium-sized mixing bowl, stir together the nondairy milk, sweetener, flax seeds, and vanilla extract. Set aside for 5 minutes, until the flax seeds absorb some of the liquid and thicken, then stir in the pumpkin puree and coconut oil.

- In a small bowl, whisk together the soy flour, coconut flour, cinnamon, baking powder, baking soda, and salt.

- Stir the dry ingredients into the pumpkin mixture until completely combined and smooth, then scoop the batter into the lined pan and spread evenly. The batter will be too thick to pour, but still loose enough to spread.

- Bake for 50 minutes, until a knife inserted in the center of the loaf comes out clean. Let the bread cool in the pan for 5 minutes before removing using the overhanging parchment as handles.

- Let cool completely before slicing.

Variation PUMPKIN MUFFINS. *Follow the recipe as written, but scoop the batter into 8 lined wells of a standard-sized muffin pan and bake for 30 minutes, until a knife inserted in the center of a muffin comes out clean. Let cool for 5 minutes before removing.*

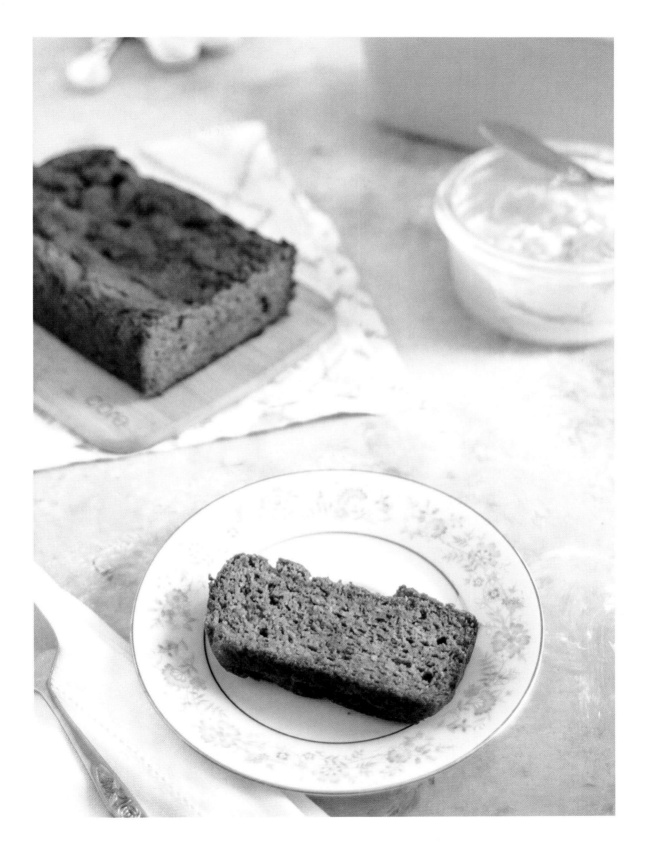

Seed Bread

This bread has rapidly become a regular breakfast item of mine. It reminds me of the dense loaves of German-style seeded rye bread that I used to love so much, back in the days when I ate lots carbohydrates and gluten. This bread is an ideal breakfast option because it's loaded with fat and protein to keep you full and energized. It also makes the perfect base for Avocado Toast (page 76).

  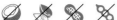

YIELD: one 9 by 5-inch (23 by 12.75-cm) loaf (12 servings)
PREP TIME: 10 minutes   COOK TIME: 1½ hours

1 cup (120g) raw pepitas (pumpkin seeds)

1 cup (120g) raw sunflower seeds

¼ cup (40g) chia seeds

½ cup (56g) pea protein powder (see Note)

¼ cup (20g) psyllium husks

½ teaspoon salt

1 cup (240 ml) water

¼ cup (64g) tahini, room temperature

- Preheat the oven to 375°F (190°C) and line a 9 by 5-inch (23 by 12.75-cm) loaf pan with parchment paper. Leave at least 2 inches (5 cm) of extra parchment on each long side of the pan for easier removal of the loaf.

- In a medium-sized mixing bowl, whisk together the seeds, protein powder, psyllium husks, and salt.

- In a small bowl or large measuring cup, stir together the water and tahini.

- Pour the tahini mixture over the seed mixture and stir until thoroughly combined and no dry spots remain. The dough will thicken as you stir and will become quite dense.

- Scoop the dough into the lined loaf pan, spread evenly, and smooth the top.

- Bake for 85 to 90 minutes, until the crust is hard and sounds hollow when tapped.

- Remove the bread from the pan using the overhanging parchment as handles and transfer to a cooling rack. Let cool completely before slicing.

To store **Store covered at room temperature for up to 3 days, refrigerate for up to a week, or slice and freeze for up to a month.**

To reheat **Place frozen slices in a preheated 350°F (177°C) oven for about 5 minutes, until warmed through, or for up to 10 minutes to toast them.**

Note **Pea protein yields the best results in this recipe. Some protein powders (like soy isolate) do not work the same way.**

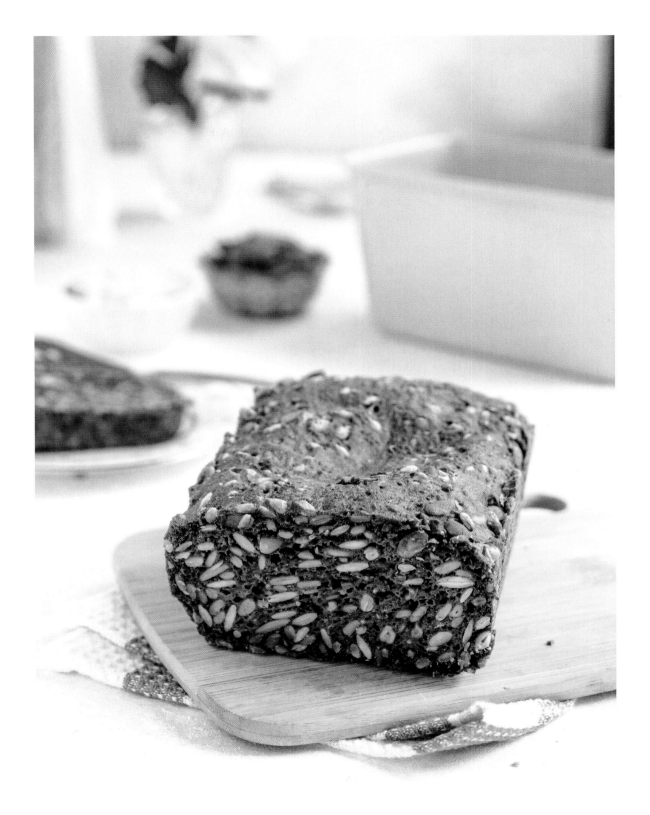

Avocado Toast

It's easy to understand how avocado toast became so popular. There's something magical about a nice piece of crunchy toast topped with creamy avocado and fresh greens, sprouts, or other veggies. I love topping mine with broccoli sprouts to add some liver-supporting sulfur compounds to my day, along with the B vitamins in the avocado.

  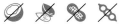

YIELD: 2 servings   PREP TIME: 5 minutes (not including time to make bread)   COOK TIME: 5 minutes

4 thick slices Seed Bread (page 74)

1 medium Hass avocado (7½ ounces/212g)

1 tablespoon lime or lemon juice

1 teaspoon crushed garlic

Salt

Ground black pepper

SUGGESTED TOPPINGS:

Microgreens

Broccoli sprouts

Sliced radishes

Sliced tomatoes

Sliced scallions (green parts only)

Everything Bagel Blend (page 174)

- Preheat the oven to 300°F (150°C).

- Place the slices of bread directly on the oven rack and bake for 5 minutes, or until slightly toasted. Remove the toast from the oven.

- Cut the avocado in half, remove the pit, and scoop the flesh into a small mixing bowl. Add the lime juice and garlic and mash until the ingredients are evenly distributed.

- Divide the avocado mixture evenly among the pieces of toast, sprinkle with salt and pepper to taste, and top as desired.

To store **Refrigerate the bread, avocado mixture, and toppings separately in tightly sealed containers for up to 2 days.**

NUTRITION INFORMATION (without toppings): **501** calories | **39.8g** fat | **22.4g** protein | **20.5g** total carbs | **7.1g** net carbs

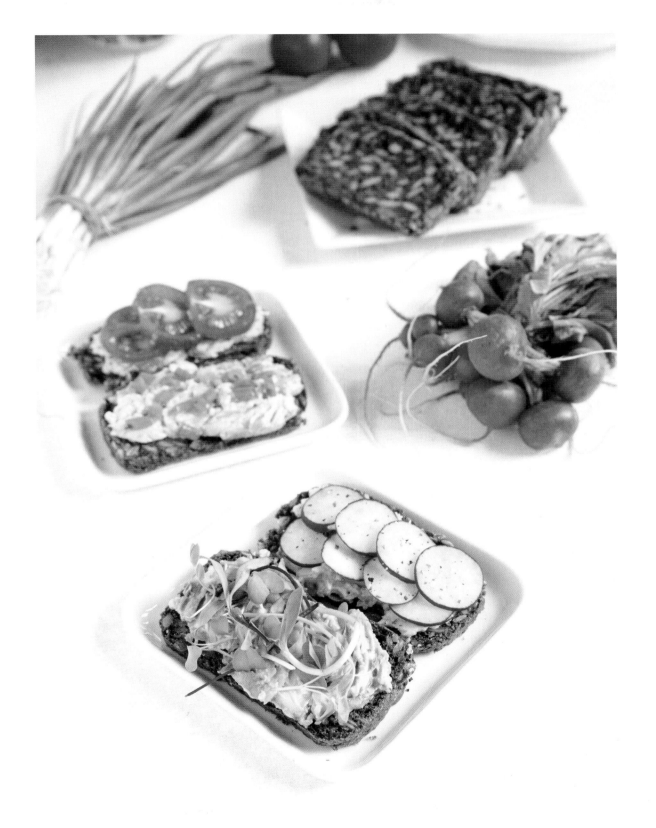

Chia Pudding Three Ways

It took me a while to warm up to chia pudding, but eventually I got there, and now it's a breakfast staple for me—especially when I'm short on time in the morning or I need to grab something on the go. These puddings are a great way to add protein, fiber, and anti-inflammatory omega-3 fatty acids to your diet.

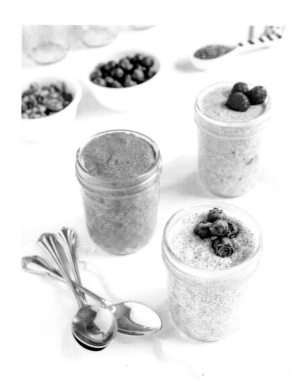

Basic Chia Pudding

¾ cup (180 ml) unsweetened coconut milk or other nondairy milk of choice

3 tablespoons (30g) chia seeds

¼ teaspoon vanilla extract

8 to 10 drops liquid stevia (optional)

SUGGESTED TOPPINGS:

Berries

Unsweetened coconut flakes

To store **Refrigerate in a tightly sealed jar for up to 3 days.**

YIELD: 1 serving   PREP TIME: 5 minutes, plus 10 minutes to thicken

- Put all the ingredients in a jar that holds at least 8 fluid ounces (240 ml). Secure the lid tightly and shake until well combined. Let the mixture sit for 10 minutes, until the chia seeds have absorbed almost all of the coconut milk.

- Stir to break up any clumps, top with berries or coconut flakes, if desired, and enjoy.

NUTRITION INFORMATION (not including toppings): **178** calories | **12.6g** fat | **5.3g** protein | **7.2g** total carbs | **4g** net carbs

Almond Butter & Raspberry Chia Pudding

²/₃ cup (160 ml) unsweetened almond milk or other nondairy milk of choice

2 tablespoons (32g) unsweetened creamy almond butter, room temperature

1 tablespoon frozen raspberries or 5 fresh raspberries

3 tablespoons (30g) chia seeds

8 to 10 drops liquid stevia (optional)

SUGGESTED TOPPINGS:

More raspberries

YIELD: 1 serving   PREP TIME: 5 minutes, plus 10 minutes to thicken

- Put half of the milk and the almond butter in a jar that holds at least 8 fluid ounces (240 ml). With a fork, whisk until the almond butter is dissolved. Add the raspberries and use the fork to break them up.

- Add the chia seeds, stevia, and the rest of the almond milk. Secure the lid tightly and shake until well combined. Let the mixture sit for 10 minutes, until the chia seeds have absorbed almost all of the milk.

- Stir to break up any clumps, top with more raspberries, and enjoy.

To store **Refrigerate in a tightly sealed jar for up to 3 days.**

NUTRITION INFORMATION (not including toppings): **411** calories | **33.9g** fat | **14g** protein | **19.2g** total carbs | **6.3g** net carbs

Silky Smooth Chocolate Chia Pudding

¾ cup (180 ml) unsweetened coconut milk or other nondairy milk of choice

3 tablespoons (30g) chia seeds

1 rounded tablespoon cocoa powder

8 to 10 drops liquid stevia (optional)

SUGGESTED TOPPINGS:

Berries

Unsweetened coconut flakes

To store **Refrigerate in a tightly sealed jar for up to 3 days.**

YIELD: 1 serving   PREP TIME: 5 minutes

- Put all the ingredients in a blender or food processor and blend until smooth, about 2 minutes. The pudding will have thickened considerably but should still be pourable. If the pudding is too thick to pour, blend in 1 tablespoon of coconut milk at a time until the desired consistency is reached.

- To serve, pour into a bowl or jar that holds at least 8 fluid ounces (240 ml) and top with berries or coconut flakes, if desired.

NUTRITION INFORMATION (not including toppings): **190** calories | **13.3g** fat | **6.4g** protein | **16.4g** total carbs | **3.9g** net carbs

Tahini Bagels

When I first started out on a ketogenic diet, I missed bagels terribly. Arriving at this recipe was well worth the trial and error. While these bagels don't taste exactly like the real thing, they're a delicious substitute that hits the spot. This is one of the most popular recipes on my blog, and it has gone through quite a few evolutions thanks to all of the feedback from my readers. This iteration is the newest and most improved. While these bagels are delicious plain, they are even better with some Everything Bagel Blend on top!

   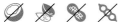

½ cup (56g) ground flax seeds

¼ cup (20g) psyllium husks

¾ teaspoon baking powder

¼ teaspoon salt

1 cup (240 ml) warm water

½ cup (132g) tahini, room temperature

TOPPINGS (OPTIONAL):

Sesame seeds

Everything Bagel Blend (page 174)

Keto Buttery Spread (page 187) or vegan butter substitute of choice

To store: Keep in a covered container on the counter for up to 3 days or freeze for up to a month.

To reheat: Place frozen bagels in a preheated 300°F (150°C) oven for about 5 minutes, until warmed through. If you want to toast the bagels, slice the warmed bagel in half and return it to the oven for another 5 minutes.

YIELD: 6 bagels (1 per serving)
PREP TIME: 10 minutes COOK TIME: 40 minutes

- Preheat the oven to 375°F (190°C) and grease a standard-size 6-well doughnut pan or line a rimmed baking sheet with parchment paper.

- In a small mixing bowl, whisk together the flax seeds, psyllium husks, baking powder, and salt.

- In a separate small bowl, whisk together the water and tahini.

- Stir the dry ingredients into the wet ingredients, then knead to form a dough. The dough will be thick and sticky.

- To make the bagels in a doughnut pan, press the dough into the greased wells of the doughnut pan, making sure to distribute it evenly.

  To make the bagels on a baking sheet, divide the dough into 6 equal-sized balls. Use your hands to form each ball into a disc that is about 4 inches (10 cm) in diameter and ¼ inch (6 mm) thick. Poke a hole in the center of each disc with your finger and stretch until the hole is about 1 inch (2.5 cm) in diameter. Lay the bagels on the parchment-lined baking sheet.

- If desired, sprinkle the bagels with sesame seeds or Everything Bagel Blend before baking.

- Bake for about 40 minutes, until golden brown. Let cool completely on the pan before removing.

- To enjoy, cut a bagel in half and toast like you would a normal bagel. Then top as desired!

NUTRITION INFORMATION (without toppings): **209** calories | **16.4g** fat | **6.6g** protein | **9.4g** total carbs | **2g** net carbs

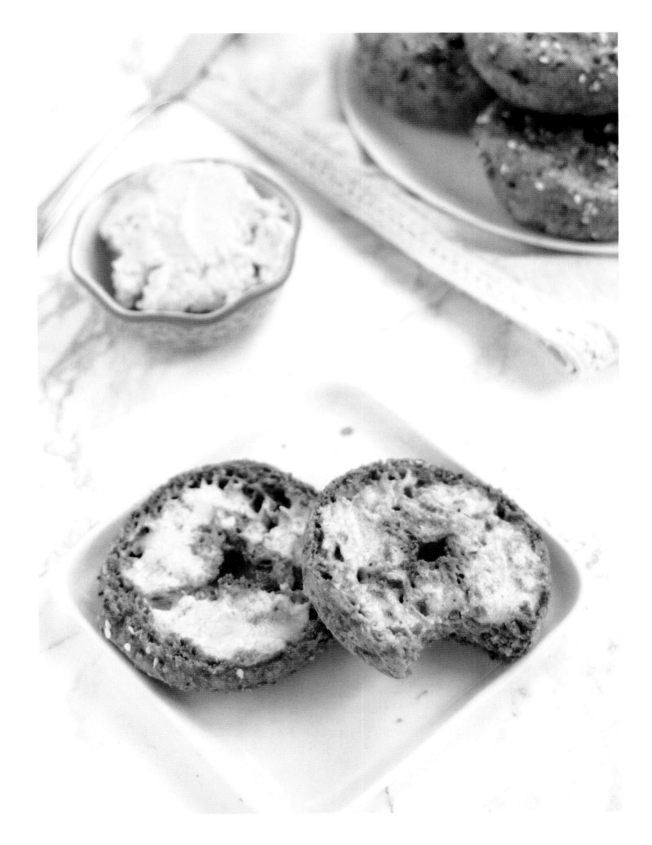

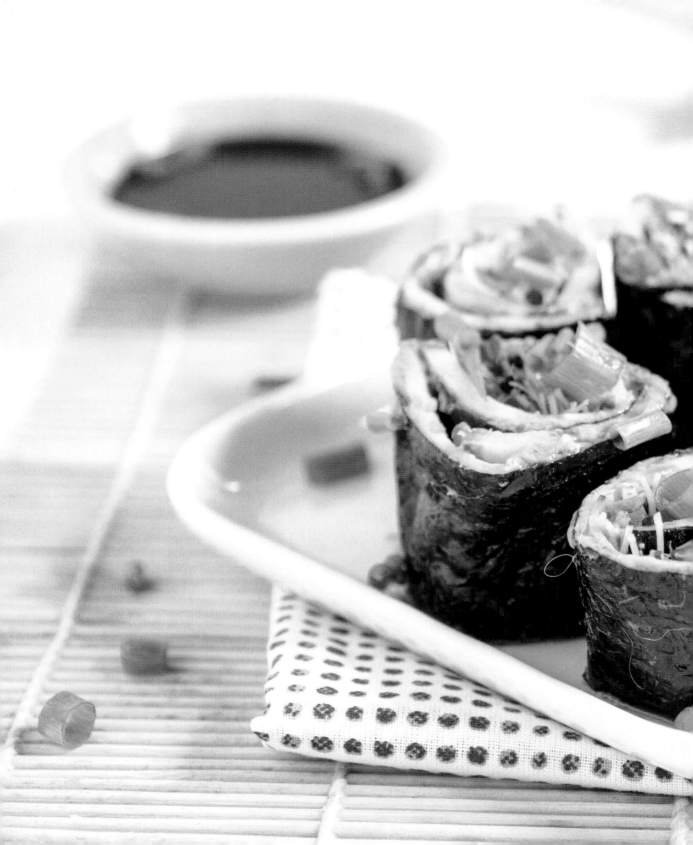

Snacks

Coco-Nutty Trail Mix

One of my absolute favorite activities is hiking through the White Mountains in New Hampshire. All-day hikes require a lot of portable food, so I always pack some trail mix. I've also been known to eat this like cereal with coconut milk.

While the freeze-dried berries are optional, they add tartness and flavor; leave them out to reduce the net carbs by 0.7 gram per serving.

YIELD: about 4 cups (255g) (about ⅔ cup/40g per serving)
PREP TIME: 5 minutes   COOK TIME: 10 minutes

1 cup (60g) unsweetened coconut flakes

1 cup (120g) chopped raw pecans

½ cup (60g) raw pepitas (pumpkin seeds)

¼ cup (30g) cacao nibs

¼ cup (7g) freeze-dried raspberries or strawberries (optional)

- Preheat the oven to 300°F (150°C).

- Spread the coconut, pecans, and pepitas on a rimmed baking sheet and toast in the oven for 10 minutes, until the coconut flakes turn a light golden brown.

- Remove from the oven and let cool completely before mixing in the cacao nibs and freeze-dried berries.

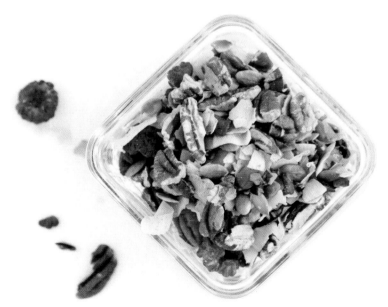

To store **Keep in a tightly sealed jar at room temperature for up to a week.**

NUTRITION INFORMATION: **211** calories | **19.9g** fat | **5.2g** protein | **7.7g** total carbs | **2.7g** net carbs

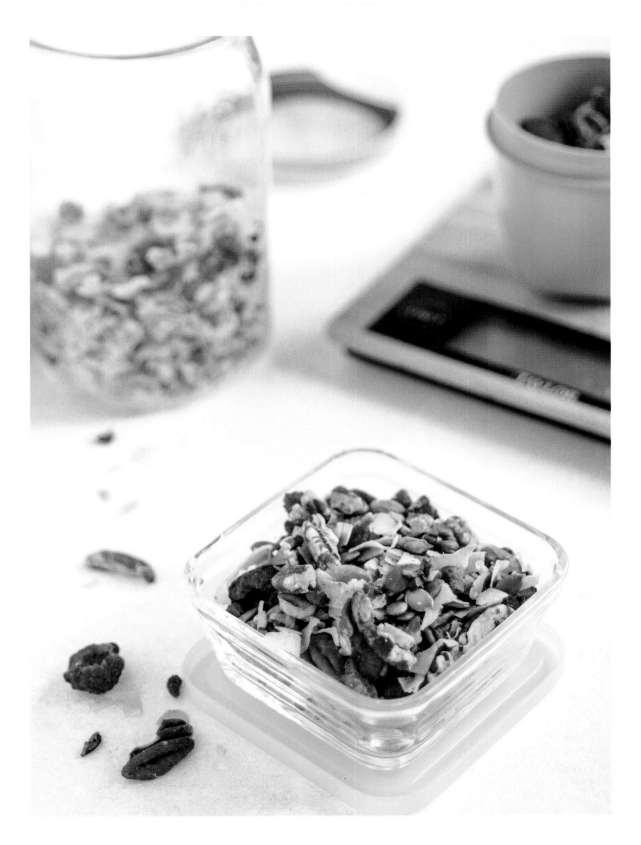

Baked Radish Chips

There seems to be a trendy new veggie chip every time I turn around, but I have always found radish chips to be the tastiest. Radishes add their own bite that makes these chips a bit more exciting than other veggie varieties. Any type of radish will do, from daikon to watermelon to the typical French breakfast radish commonly sold in supermarkets, which is what I used here. While slicing the radishes with a knife is certainly an option, using a mandoline slicer saves both time and effort here.

   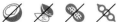

YIELD: 4 servings   PREP TIME: 15 minutes   COOK TIME: 25 minutes

1 pound (454g) large radishes, thinly sliced

½ teaspoon salt

¼ cup (60 ml) extra-virgin olive oil

¼ teaspoon granulated garlic

¼ teaspoon cracked black pepper

- Preheat the oven to 375°F (190°C) and line a rimmed baking sheet with parchment paper.

- In a large mixing bowl, toss the radish slices with the salt. Let sit for 5 minutes.

- After 5 minutes, the radishes should have released some moisture. Spread the radish slices on a clean dish towel or paper towel and blot dry. Dry the mixing bowl.

- Return the radishes to the mixing bowl and add the olive oil, granulated garlic, and pepper. Mix to coat the radishes in the oil and spices.

- Arrange the radishes on the lined baking sheet so that they do not overlap.

- Bake for 25 minutes, until the larger chips are uniformly golden. Serve warm.

To store Refrigerate in a tightly sealed container for up to 3 days.

To reheat Spread the chips in a thin layer on a rimmed baking sheet and heat in a preheated 300°F (150°C) oven for 5 minutes, until warmed.

NUTRITION INFORMATION: **138** calories | **13.6g** fat | **0.8g** protein | **4g** total carbs | **2g** net carbs

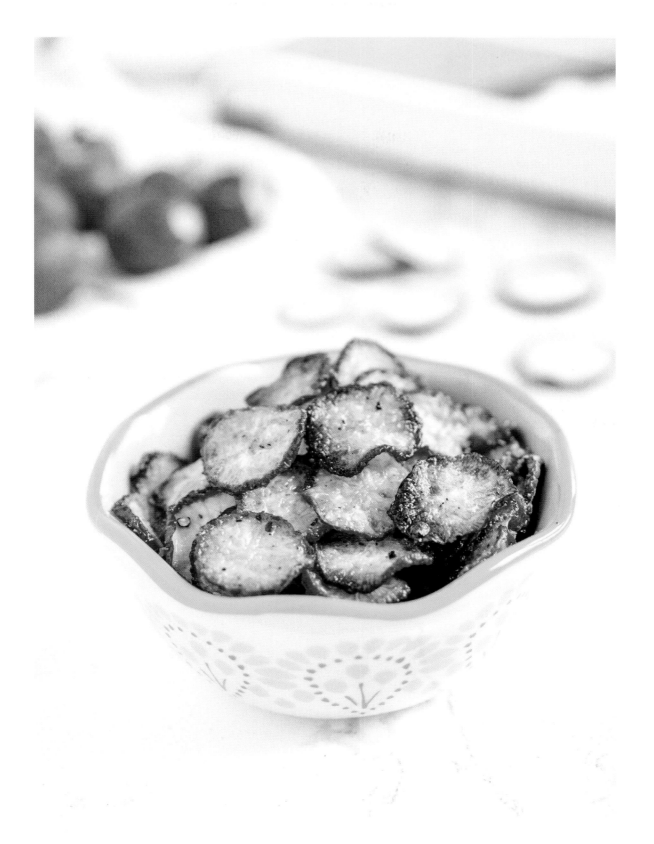

No-Cook Falafel

Falafel is one of my favorite foods, a preference that formed while I was living across from a falafel place that stayed open until 2am. Even though I haven't lived near that restaurant for almost a decade, I still crave falafel more than any other food. Keto falafel is a challenge to pull off, as chickpeas are a little too high in carbs. I like to use hemp seeds as a stand-in for this recipe; they provide protein and omega-3 fatty acids with minimal carbohydrates. These falafel balls require no cooking and are delicious as a snack dipped in Tahini Dressing (page 186) or as part of a Falafel Salad (page 106).

YIELD: 10 balls (1 per serving)   PREP TIME: 10 minutes, plus time to chill

¾ cup (120g) hulled hemp seeds

1 tablespoon dried parsley leaves

1½ teaspoons ground cumin

1 teaspoon granulated onion

½ teaspoon granulated garlic

¼ teaspoon cracked black pepper

Grated zest of 1 lemon

¼ cup (64g) tahini, room temperature

• Line a rimmed baking sheet with parchment paper.

• Using a food processor or blender, grind the hemp seeds until a coarse meal forms.

• Transfer the hemp meal to a medium-sized mixing bowl, then add the rest of ingredients except the tahini and whisk together until combined.

• Stir in the tahini and continue to mix until the ingredients are well combined and a somewhat crumbly dough forms. It will have the texture of pie dough and should hold together when pinched.

• Using your hands, roll the mixture into 10 balls, about 1 tablespoon each. Place the balls on the lined baking sheet.

• Chill in the freezer for at least 30 minutes or in the refrigerator for 2 hours so the falafel balls hold together.

To store Refrigerate in a tightly sealed container for up to a week or freeze for up to a month.

NUTRITION INFORMATION: **106** calories | **9.1g** fat | **5.4g** protein | **2.4g** total carbs | **1.2g** net carbs

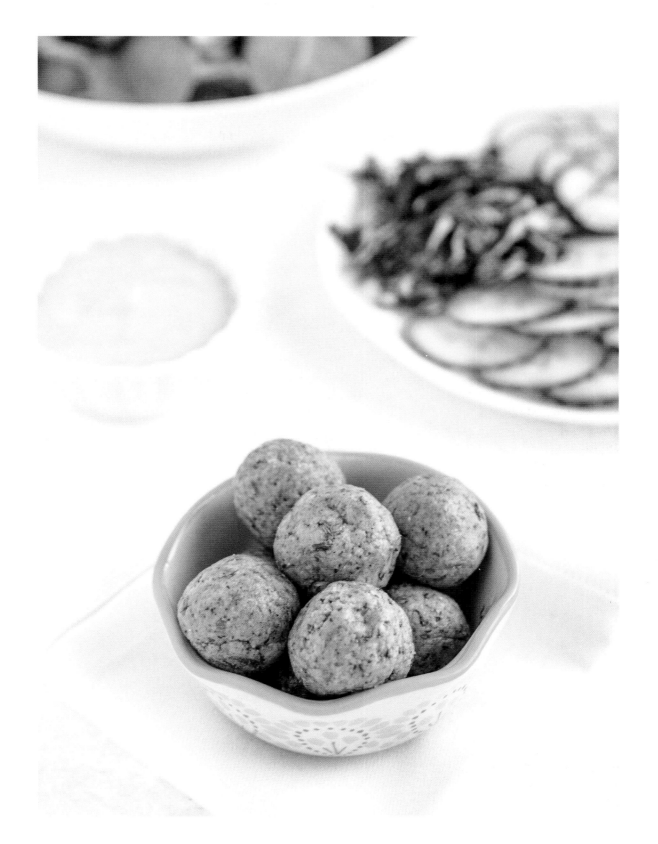

Flaxitos

In reality, these are just slightly gussied-up flax crackers, but I like to call them Flaxitos as a tribute to the tortilla chips that I inhaled as a teenager. This recipe is really simple and versatile—you can add 1 tablespoon of pretty much any seasoning you'd like to the base recipe to vary the flavor profile. Two of my favorite additions are chili powder and za'atar.

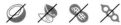

YIELD: 6 servings   PREP TIME: 5 minutes, plus 20 minutes to cool
COOK TIME: 35 minutes

1 cup (112g) ground flax seeds

¼ cup (20g) nutritional yeast

1 teaspoon granulated garlic

½ teaspoon salt

¾ cup (180 ml) water

- Preheat the oven to 350°F (177°C) and line a rimmed baking sheet with parchment paper.

- In a medium-sized mixing bowl, mix together the flax seeds, nutritional yeast, granulated garlic, and salt until the ingredients are evenly distributed.

- Pour in the water and stir for about a minute, until a thick batter forms. It should be spreadable and have the texture of natural peanut butter. If it's too thick to spread, stir in a little more water.

- Spread the dough in a thin layer on the lined baking sheet and use the back of a spoon to smooth it out. Use a butter knife to score the dough into triangle shapes.

- Bake for 35 minutes, until the crackers are firm to the touch and there are no soft spots remaining.

- Remove from the oven and let cool for about 20 minutes so that the crackers set up. Break apart before serving.

To store **Keep in a tightly sealed container at room temperature for up to 4 days.**

NUTRITION INFORMATION: **106** calories | **9.1g** fat | **3g** protein | **2.4g** total carbs | **1.2g** net carbs

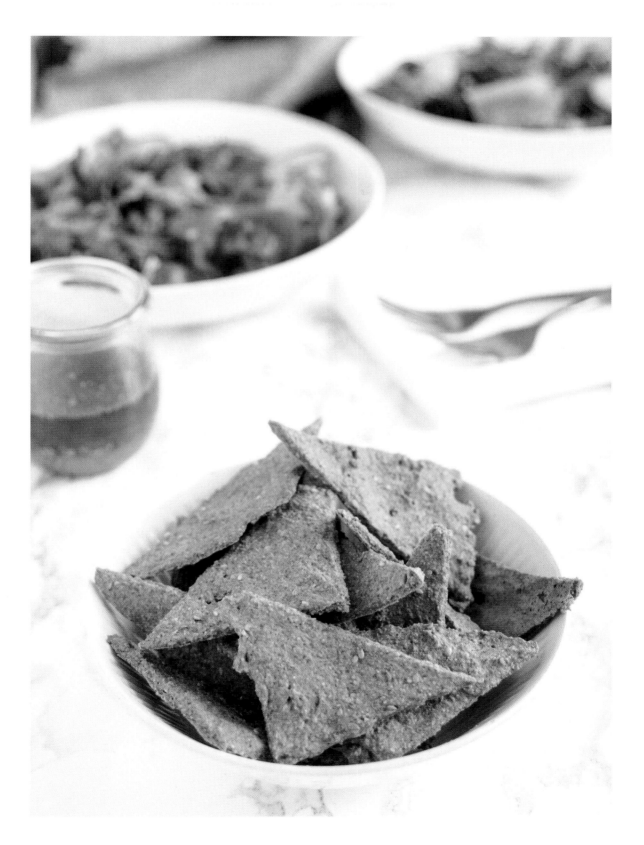

Garlic Dill Kale Chips

I love kale chips, but most commercial brands are pretty high in carbs. Some even contain agave nectar or maple syrup! Fortunately, this version is totally keto-friendly, and I think these chips are even tastier than a lot of the store-bought varieties.

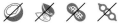

YIELD: 4 servings   PREP TIME: 10 minutes   COOK TIME: 18 minutes

¼ cup plus 2 tablespoons (96g) tahini, room temperature

2 tablespoons (30 ml) extra-virgin olive oil

1 tablespoon apple cider vinegar

1 tablespoon crushed garlic

½ teaspoon salt

¼ packed cup (5g) fresh dill leaves, finely chopped

2 packed cups (140g) destemmed and chopped kale

- Preheat the oven to 375°F (190°C) and line a rimmed baking sheet with parchment paper.

- In a large mixing bowl, whisk together the tahini, olive oil, vinegar, garlic, and salt until well combined. Stir in the dill.

- Add the kale and toss with the tahini mixture until well coated. It's helpful to use your hands and really massage the dressing into the leaves.

- Spread the kale in a thin layer on the lined baking sheet and bake for 18 minutes, until the kale chips are uniformly crispy and dry.

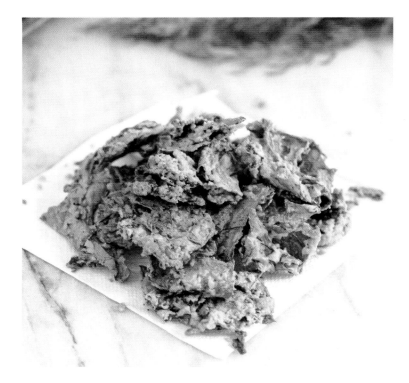

To store Keep in a tightly sealed container at room temperature for up to 1 day.

To recrisp If the air is humid and the chips become soggy, bake them at 300°F (150°C) for 5 minutes, until they are crispy again.

NUTRITION INFORMATION: **208** calories | **18.9g** fat | **5.4g** protein | **7.6g** total carbs | **4.3g** net carbs

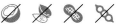

Lupini Hummus

Hummus is one of those foods that I could happily eat off of a spoon all day long. Unfortunately, chickpeas are a little higher in carbs than I would like. While chickpea hummus certainly can have a place in a keto diet, this version made with lupini beans has a much more favorable carb count. It has half the net carbs of traditional hummus, so you can eat twice as much for the same carb count. What's not to love about that?

YIELD: 2½ cups (600 ml) (¼ cup/60 ml per serving)
PREP TIME: 5 minutes

1½ cups (250g) jarred lupini beans (packed in brine), drained

½ cup (120 ml) extra-virgin olive oil

½ cup (120 ml) water

¼ cup (64g) tahini, room temperature

Juice of 1 lemon

1 teaspoon crushed garlic

1 teaspoon ground cumin

Paprika, for sprinkling

Put the lupini beans, olive oil, water, tahini, lemon juice, garlic, and cumin in a food processor or high-powered blender and blend until smooth, 2 to 3 minutes. Transfer to a serving bowl and sprinkle with paprika.

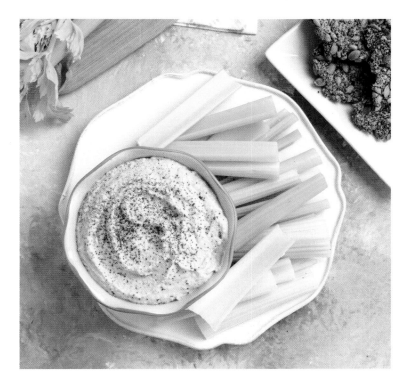

To store Refrigerate in a tightly sealed container for up to 4 days.

NUTRITION INFORMATION: **162** calories | **14.7g** fat | **5g** protein | **4g** total carbs | **2.7g** net carbs

Seed Crackers

Sometimes you just want something crunchy and a little bit salty. These seed crackers not only bring crunch and flavor to the table but also contain a decent amount of protein and some B vitamins to boot! I like the combination of pepitas and sunflower seeds, but if you want to reduce the carb count even further, you can use 1 cup (120g) of pepitas and omit the sunflower seeds.

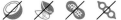

YIELD: about 30 crackers (2 by 3 inches/5 by 7.5 cm each; 5 crackers per serving)
PREP TIME: 10 minutes   COOK TIME: 30 minutes

½ cup (80g) chia seeds

½ cup (60g) raw pepitas (pumpkin seeds)

½ cup (60g) raw sunflower seeds

2 tablespoons (32g) tahini, room temperature

¾ cup (180 ml) water

1 tablespoon dehydrated onion flakes

¼ teaspoon salt

- Preheat the oven to 350°F (177°C) and line a rimmed baking sheet with parchment paper.

- In a medium-sized mixing bowl, stir together all the ingredients. Let sit for about 10 minutes, until the chia seeds have absorbed all of the water and a thick dough forms.

- Spread the dough in a thin layer (no more than ¼ inch/ 5 mm) on the lined baking sheet and use the back of a spoon to smooth it out.

- Bake for 30 minutes, until the crackers are uniformly dry and lightly golden.

- Remove from the oven and let cool before breaking apart.

To store **Store in an airtight container at room temperature for up to 4 days.**

Note **For a more uniform look, score the crackers into 2 by 3-inch (5 by 7.5-cm) pieces before baking.**

NUTRITION INFORMATION: **208** calories | **16.4g** fat | **8g** protein | **10.5g** total carbs | **3.9g** net carbs

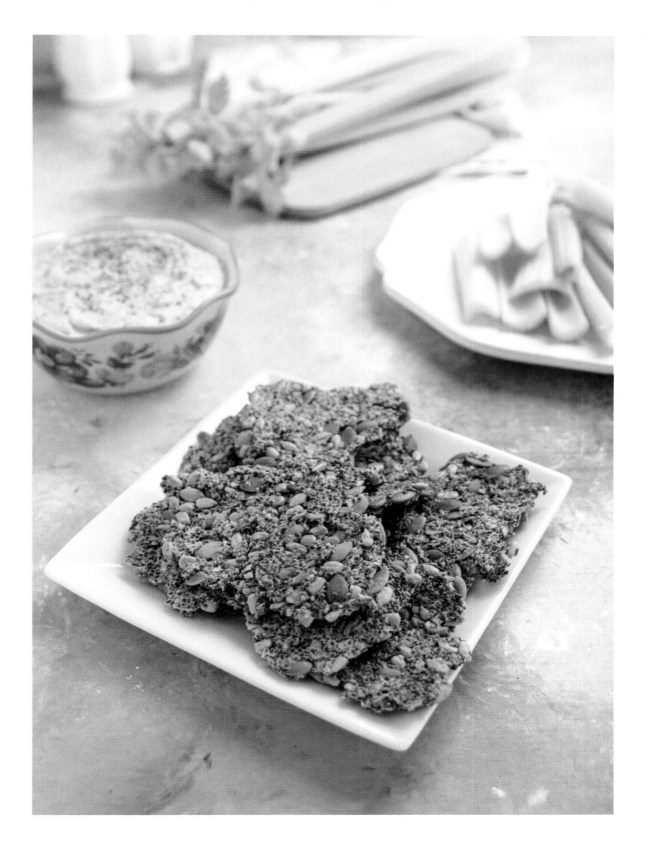

Nori Energy Sticks

These nori sticks are a homemade version of a snack that I used to buy all the time when I worked at a health food store. I really like the way they "snap" when you bite into them. I usually bring a few of these with me on long trips or casual hikes, as they are portable and aren't as messy as trail mix.

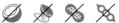

YIELD: 12 sticks (2 per serving)
PREP TIME: 15 minutes   COOK TIME: 45 minutes

4 sheets sushi nori

1 cup (120g) raw sunflower seeds

2 tablespoons (20g) chia seeds

1 tablespoon chili powder or curry powder

¼ teaspoon salt

¼ cup (60 ml) water

- Preheat the oven to 180°F (82°C) and line a rimmed baking sheet with parchment. Prepare a small dish of water for sealing the nori sheets.

- Cut the nori sheets into thirds using kitchen shears.

- In a food processor, grind the sunflower seeds into a flour.

- In a small mixing bowl, stir together the sunflower seed flour, chia seeds, chili powder, salt, and water until a thick dough forms. It should hold its shape when pinched.

- Lay out one of your cut pieces of nori and place 1½ tablespoons of the seed mixture in a line, lengthwise down the piece of nori. Using your fingers, lightly wet the outside edge of the nori. Starting with the inside edge, roll the nori tightly around the seed mixture and seal the roll shut by pressing the wet side of the nori. Place the nori roll on the baking sheet, seam side down. Repeat until the seed mixture is used up; you should have 12 nori sticks.

- Bake the nori sticks for 45 minutes, until they are firm and dry to the touch. Let cool before storing.

To store **Place in a ventilated container (such as a paper bag) for up to 3 days.**

NUTRITION INFORMATION: **163** calories | **13.3g** fat | **6.4g** protein | **7.5g** total carbs | **3.2g** net carbs

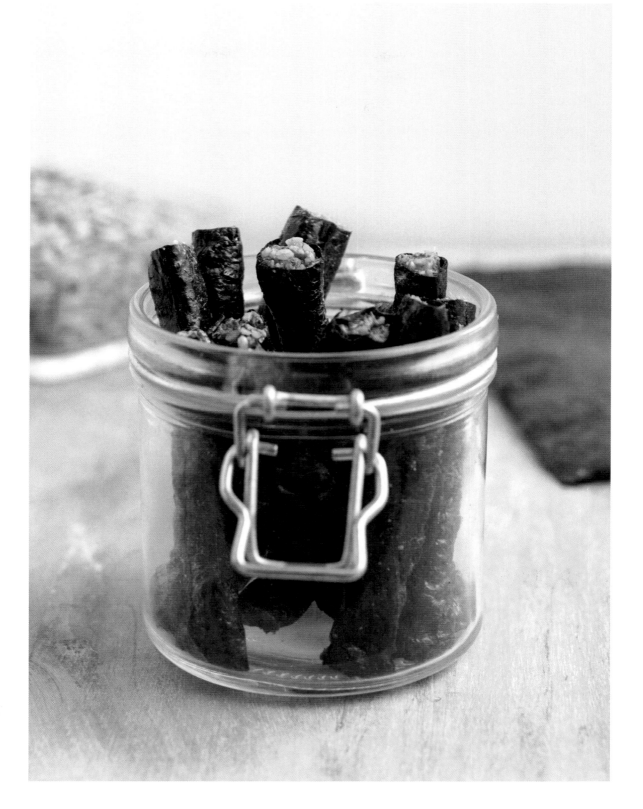

Easy Peanut Butter Protein Bars

Sometimes it's nice to have a convenient snack to grab on the go, and these protein bars really fit the bill for me. I'll pop one or two in my bag in the morning if I'm going to be out for a while so I have a keto-friendly snack on hand. If you don't eat peanut butter, almond butter or sunflower seed butter works equally well.

YIELD: 6 bars (1 per serving)   PREP TIME: 10 minutes, plus 1 hour to chill

1 tablespoon ground flax seeds

½ cup (120 ml) pea milk or other nondairy milk of choice

2 tablespoons (24g) granulated sweetener, powdered (see Note)

½ cup (128g) unsweetened creamy peanut butter, room temperature

½ cup (56g) pea protein powder or other vegan protein powder of choice

¼ cup (30g) cacao nibs

- Line a 9 by 5-inch (23 by 12.75-cm) loaf pan with parchment paper.

- In a large mixing bowl, whisk together the flax seeds, nondairy milk, and sweetener. Add the peanut butter and protein powder and stir until a thick dough forms. Knead the dough until it is uniform.

- Press the dough into the lined loaf pan and sprinkle the cacao nibs on top. Gently press the cacao nibs into the dough so they stick.

- Refrigerate for at least an hour, until the bars have firmed up somewhat, then slice and serve.

To store Refrigerate in a tightly sealed container for up to 3 days.

Note I don't buy a separate powdered sweetener; I just weigh out granulated sweetener and then pulverize it in a coffee or spice grinder.

NUTRITION INFORMATION: **183** calories | **12.9g** fat | **14.1g** protein | **9.3g** total carbs | **2.8g** net carbs

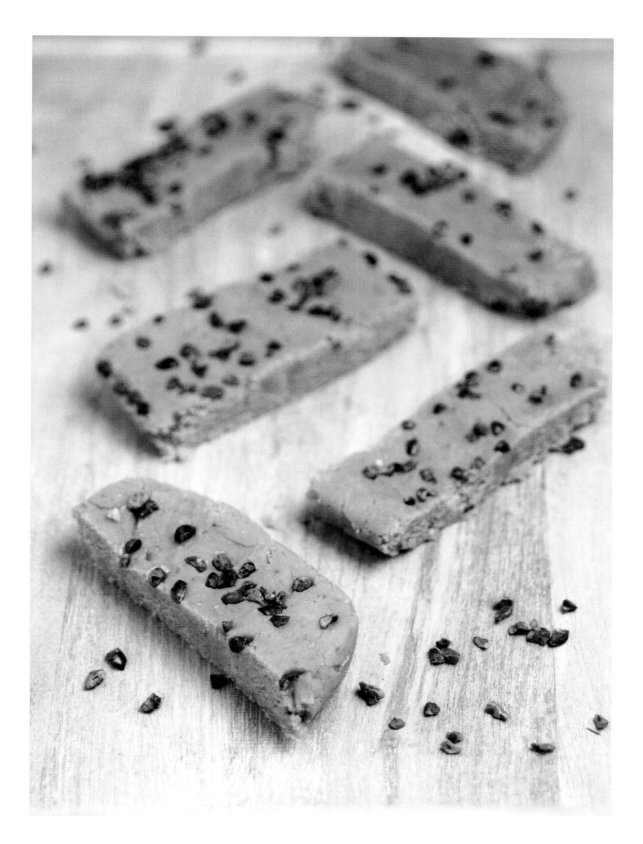

Cucumber Avocado Pinwheels

This is basically a lazy version of sushi that I used to make when my roommates and I would have a sushi night. I really like sneaking broccoli sprouts into these rolls as a way to consume those important sulfur compounds. If broccoli sprouts aren't your thing, thinly sliced red, orange, or yellow bell peppers are a delicious substitute (though a bit higher in carbs).

   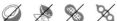

YIELD: 2 servings (6 to 8 pieces per serving) PREP TIME: 10 minutes

1 medium Hass avocado (7½ ounces/212g)

2 sheets sushi nori

2 tablespoons (20g) sesame seeds

½ cup (50g) thinly sliced cucumbers

½ cup (30g) broccoli sprouts

DIPPING SAUCE SUGGESTIONS:

Low-sodium tamari or coconut aminos with sliced scallions (green parts only)

Tangy Avocado Mayo (page 183) or vegan mayo of choice

- Cut the avocado in half and remove the pit. Scoop the flesh into a small dish and mash with a fork.

- Lay each sheet of nori on a flat surface and spread half of the mashed avocado on each sheet, leaving 1 inch (2.5 cm) of space at the far end of each sheet.

- Sprinkle a tablespoon of the sesame seeds over the avocado on each sheet.

- Lay out half of the cucumber slices on each sheet and top each with half of the broccoli sprouts.

- Wet the far edge of each nori sheet with a little water. Starting at the edge closest to you, roll up the sheet into a roll. Press gently along the seam to make sure the wet edge of nori is sealed up against the roll.

- Slice each roll into 6 to 8 pieces (depending on your preference), running the knife under water before each cut.

- Serve with the dipping sauce of your choice.

To store **Refrigerate in a tightly sealed container for up to 2 days.**

NUTRITION INFORMATION (without sauce): **201** calories | **16.4g** fat | **6.2g** protein | **10.8g** total carbs | **2.5g** net carbs

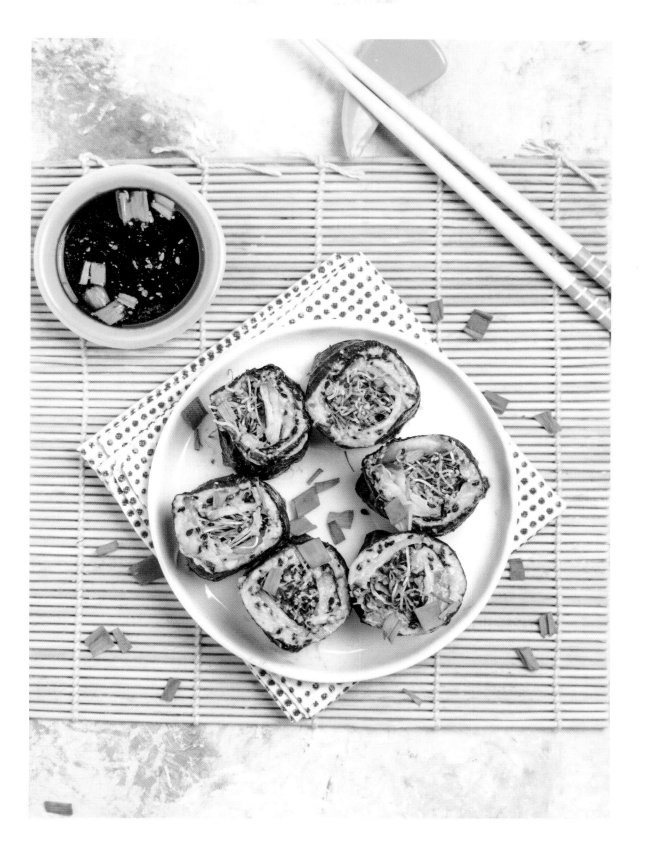

Curry Tofu Salad Bites

While these snacks can be made at any time of the year, I love to enjoy them in spring and summer. The celery and cucumber are so refreshing in warmer weather. For a hearty meal using this tofu salad, place the cucumber slices and one-quarter of the tofu salad mixture on a slice of Seed Bread (page 74) and top with some lettuce and another slice of bread.

This is another of those recipes where the flavor profile is really easy to change. I usually use a madras curry powder, but it's equally delicious made with chili powder.

YIELD: 32 bites (8 per serving)
PREP TIME: 10 minutes (not including time to make mayo)

1 (14-ounce/397-g) package extra-firm tofu, drained

¼ cup (60 ml) Tangy Avocado Mayo (page 183) or vegan mayo of choice

¼ cup (25g) diced celery

2 teaspoons curry powder or chili powder

¼ teaspoon salt

32 thin slices cucumber (about 1 cup/100g)

Cracked black pepper

2 scallions (green parts only), sliced

- In a large mixing bowl, mash together the tofu, mayo, celery, curry powder, and salt until uniformly mixed.

- Scoop about 1 tablespoon of the tofu mixture on top of each cucumber slice.

- Top with freshly ground pepper and sliced scallions and serve.

To store Refrigerate in a tightly sealed container for up to 3 days.

NUTRITION INFORMATION: **148** calories | **9.6g** fat | **11.1g** protein | **6.5g** total carbs | **3.7g** net carbs

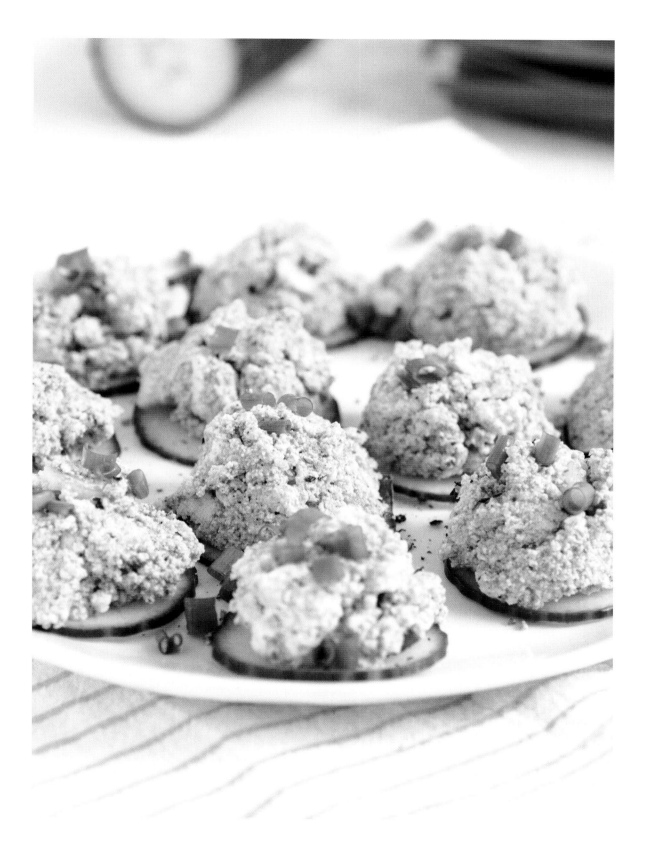

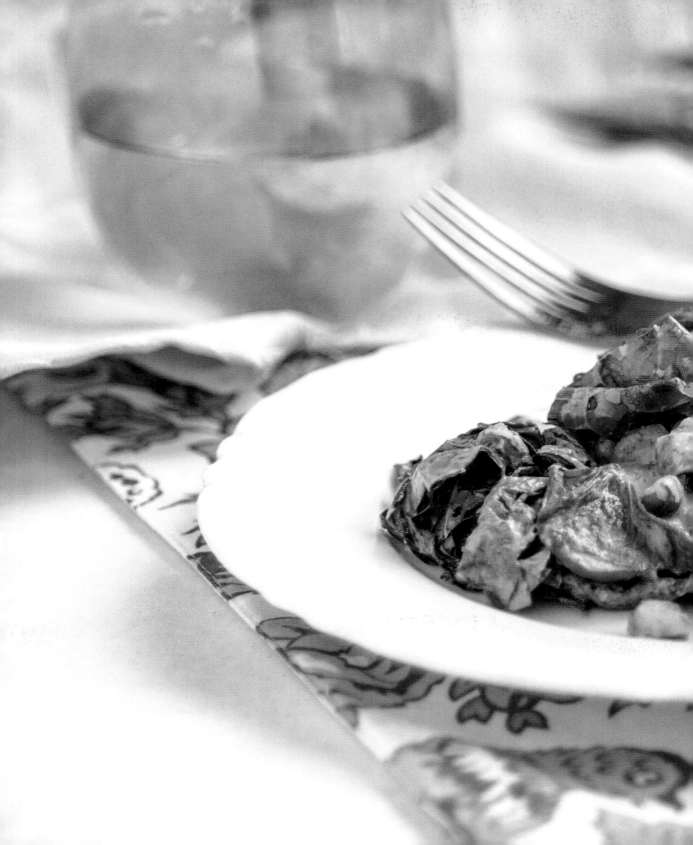

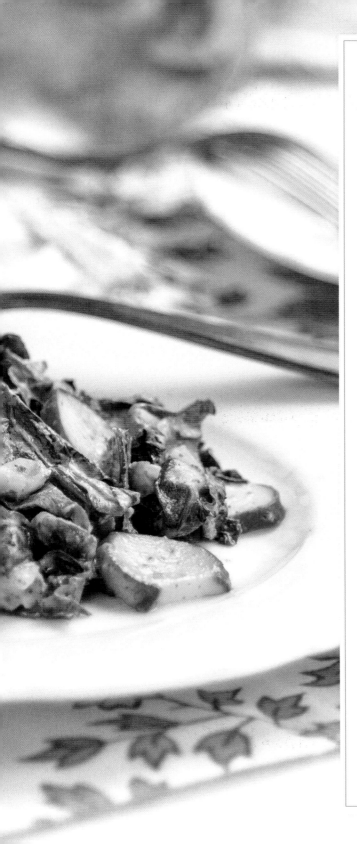

Soups, Salads & Sides

Falafel Salad

Back in the days of eating gluten, I would frequently enjoy falafel wrapped in a nice warm pita. The pita days are gone, but I do still enjoy falafel salad. This is a simplified version, using ingredients that are readily available and low in carbs. Be sure to make the falafel balls at least a half hour in advance of the salad so that they have time to set up in the freezer.

   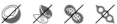

4 lightly packed cups (120g) fresh baby spinach

½ cup (60g) sliced radishes

½ cup (50g) sliced cucumbers

½ cup (30g) shredded red cabbage

1 recipe No-Cook Falafel (page 88)

¼ cup (60 ml) Tahini Dressing (page 186)

YIELD: 2 servings
PREP TIME: 10 minutes (not including time to make falafel and dressing)

- Divide the spinach, radishes, cucumbers, and cabbage between 2 bowls. Top with the falafel and dressing.

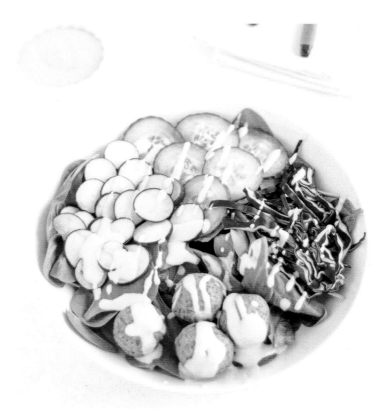

To store: *Refrigerate leftover salad separately from the falafel and dressing for up to 3 days.*

NUTRITION INFORMATION: **632** calories | **52.2g** fat | **32.4g** protein | **19.7g** total carbs | **9.8g** net carbs

Fattoush Salad

I love talking to people about food as a way to discover new flavors and dishes. This fattoush salad recipe came about when I was talking to a woman from Saudi Arabia about low-carb vegan meal options. She sent me her favorite recipe for fattoush salad and asked if I would keto-fy it for her. Since then, this has become one of my favorite salads to make. It's just so bright and flavorful!

YIELD: 4 servings   PREP TIME: 10 minutes (not including time to make Flaxitos)

DRESSING:

Juice of 1 lemon

¼ cup (60 ml) extra-virgin olive oil

1 tablespoon za'atar seasoning

¼ teaspoon granulated garlic

SALAD:

4 cups (190g) chopped romaine lettuce (about 2 hearts)

1 cup (120g) halved cherry tomatoes

1 cup (100g) sliced cucumbers

½ packed cup (30g) fresh parsley leaves, chopped

¼ packed cup (15g) fresh mint leaves, chopped

1 recipe Flaxitos (page 90)

- To make the dressing, place the ingredients in a tightly sealed jar and shake to combine.

- To make the salad, put the ingredients in a large bowl and toss to combine.

- Divide the salad among 4 serving bowls. Break one-fourth of the Flaxitos into bite-sized pieces over each bowl and top each with 2 tablespoons (30 ml) of the dressing.

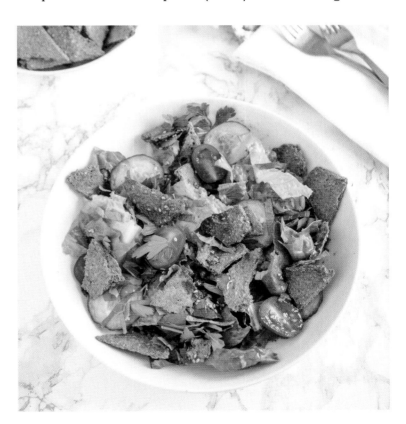

To store: *Undressed salad (without the Flaxitos) can be stored in a tightly sealed container in the refrigerator for up to 3 days. The dressing can be refrigerated for up to a week.*

Carrot Ginger Soup

Carrots are one of my favorite foods, in pretty much any form. I've been known to eat almost a half pound (over 200 grams!) of carrots in a day without giving it a second thought. So it makes sense that one of my favorite soups would be carrot based. The subtle sweetness of the carrots and coconut milk in this soup works so nicely with the punch from the ginger and the brightness of the lemon. To me, it just tastes like sunshine.

YIELD: 4 servings   PREP TIME: 5 minutes   COOK TIME: 25 minutes

2 tablespoons (30 ml) extra-virgin olive oil

1½ cups (190g) sliced carrots

1 tablespoon grated fresh ginger

1½ cups (360 ml) vegetable broth

1 (13.5-ounce/400-ml) can full-fat coconut milk

Grated zest of 1 lemon

¼ teaspoon freshly ground black pepper

- Heat the oil in a large saucepan over medium heat. Add the carrots and ginger and cook for about 5 minutes, stirring occasionally, until the carrots begin to soften.

- Add the broth and coconut milk to the pan and cover. Continue to cook for 20 minutes, until the carrots are tender and can easily be pierced with a knife.

- Pour the soup into a blender and blend until smooth, about 2 minutes.

- To serve, divide the soup among 4 bowls and top with the lemon zest and freshly ground black pepper.

To store Refrigerate in a tightly sealed container for up to 4 days or freeze for up to a month.

To reheat Warm in a covered saucepan over medium-low heat until the desired temperature is reached.

NUTRITION INFORMATION: **234** calories | **20.6g** fat | **2.1g** protein | **7.7g** total carbs | **6.3g** net carbs

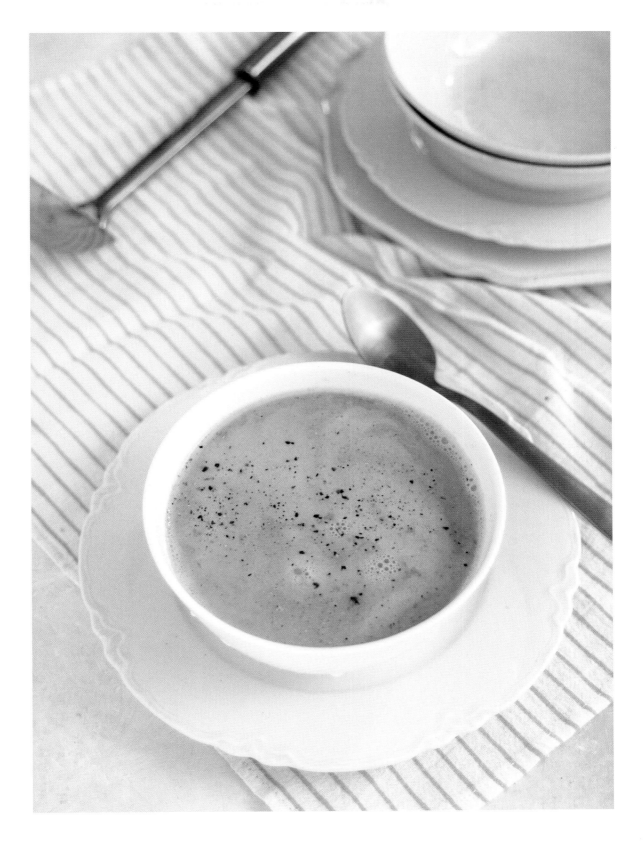

Spicy Coconut Soup

Years ago, my roommate and dear friend, Kathryn, made an incredible Thai coconut soup for me and her then-boyfriend (now husband). It was absolutely amazing, and I've been obsessed ever since. This version of the soup that she made is lower in carbs but still reminiscent of those lovely flavors.

You can make this soup soy-free by using coconut aminos rather than tamari and substituting shiitake mushrooms or a mock chicken substitute for the tofu.

YIELD: 4 servings   PREP TIME: 10 minutes   COOK TIME: 20 minutes

1 (13.5-ounce/400-ml) can full-fat coconut milk

1½ cups (350 ml) vegetable broth

1 tablespoon low-sodium tamari or coconut aminos

1 teaspoon chili paste or Sriracha sauce

1 teaspoon crushed garlic

1 teaspoon grated fresh ginger

Juice of 1 lime

1 (14-ounce/397-g) block extra-firm tofu

½ cup (50g) sliced red bell peppers, plus extra for garnish

½ cup (30g) shredded red cabbage, plus extra for garnish

FOR GARNISH (OPTIONAL):

Microgreens

1 stalk lemongrass, sliced

Grated lime zest

- Heat the coconut milk, broth, tamari, chili paste, garlic, ginger, and lime juice in a large saucepan over medium heat, stirring just to mix the ingredients, about 5 minutes.

- Drain, press, and cut the tofu into 1-inch (2.5-cm) cubes and add to the soup. Add the sliced peppers and shredded cabbage, cover, and continue to simmer for 15 minutes, until the peppers and cabbage are soft.

- Remove from the heat and portion into bowls to serve. Garnish as desired.

To store **Refrigerate in a tightly sealed container for up to 4 days or freeze for up to a month.**

To reheat **Warm in a covered saucepan over medium-low heat until the desired temperature is reached.**

NUTRITION INFORMATION (without garnishes): **162** calories | **14.7g** fat | **5g** protein | **4g** total carbs | **2.7g** net carbs

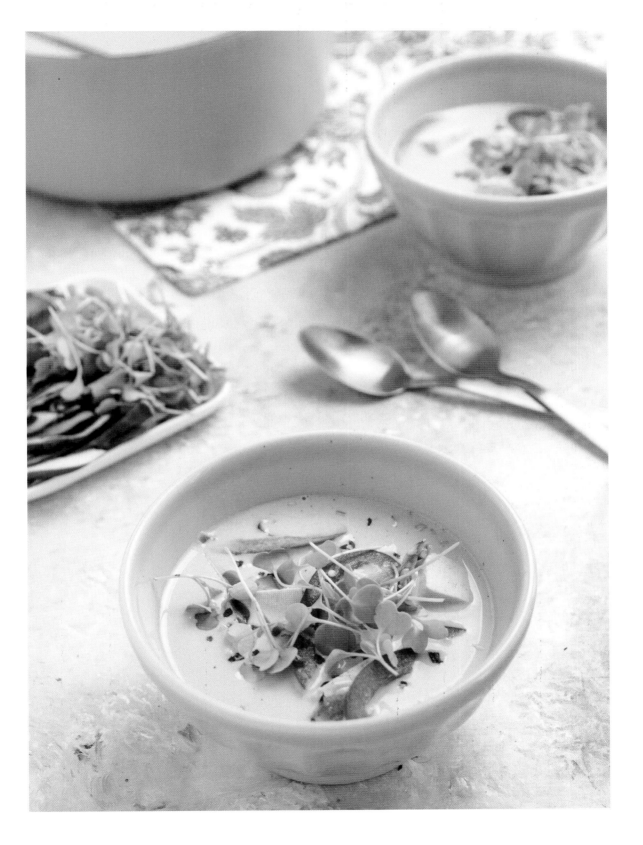

Creamy Cauliflower Soup

This recipe started out as an attempt at making a sort of faux-tato (faux potato... eh?) soup, but I decided to forgo the wordplay and let the cauliflower take center stage. The hemp seeds provide the bulk of the protein and plenty of omega-3 fatty acids, and blending them into the soup makes it super creamy.

  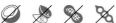

YIELD: 4 servings   PREP TIME: 5 minutes   COOK TIME: 20 minutes

2 tablespoons (30 ml) extra-virgin olive oil

4 cups (400g) cauliflower pieces

3 cups (720 ml) vegetable broth

¾ cup (120g) hulled hemp seeds

¼ cup (20g) nutritional yeast

1 tablespoon chopped fresh chives

TOPPING SUGGESTIONS:

Additional chopped fresh chives or sliced scallions (green parts only)

Sauerkraut

Freshly ground black pepper

Pinch of cayenne pepper

- Heat the oil in a large saucepan over medium heat. Add the cauliflower and cook for about 5 minutes, stirring occasionally, until the pieces begin to soften.

- Add the broth and continue to cook until the cauliflower is tender and can easily be pierced with a knife.

- Carefully pour the soup into a heat-safe high-powered blender and add the hemp seeds, nutritional yeast, and chives. Blend until smooth, 2 to 3 minutes.

- To serve, divide the soup among serving bowls and top as desired.

To store: Refrigerate in a tightly sealed container for up to 4 days or freeze for up to a month.

To reheat: Warm in a covered saucepan over medium-low heat until the desired temperature is reached.

NUTRITION INFORMATION (without toppings): **289** calories | **20.5g** fat | **16.3g** protein | **10.9g** total carbs | **3.8g** net carbs

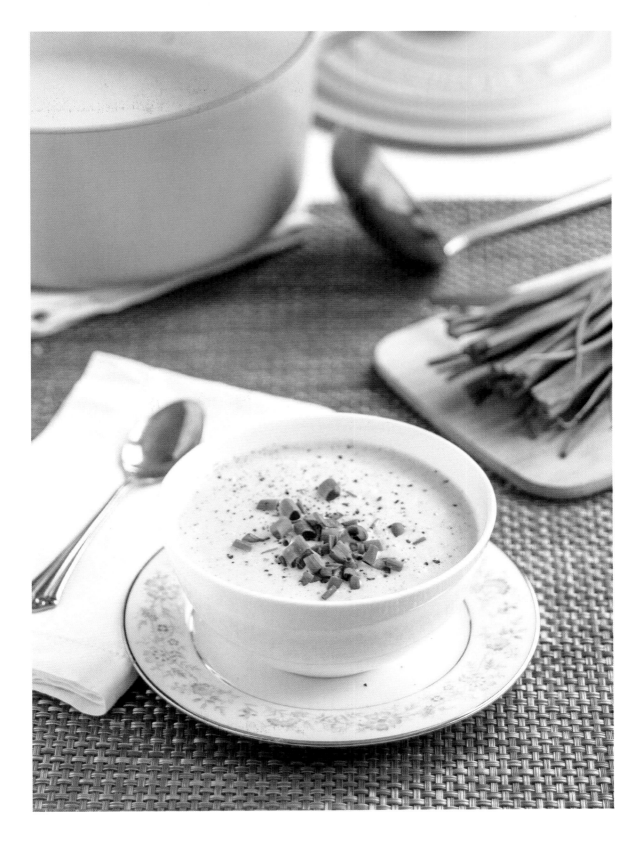

Warm Kale Salad

I live in a climate where it's not always super warm out, and in colder months, there is no way I'm going to want to eat a salad straight out of the fridge. This warm salad is perfect for those chilly spring days. It's really easy to throw together and is surprisingly flavorful for a recipe with so few ingredients.

While I most often make this salad with hazelnuts, you can easily substitute sunflower seeds or pepitas if you do not eat nuts.

YIELD: 2 servings · PREP TIME: 8 minutes (not including time to make dressing) · COOK TIME: 5 minutes

¼ cup (60 ml) Easy Mustard Vinaigrette (page 184), divided

4 cups (64g) chopped kale

2 ounces (56g) radishes, trimmed and sliced

¼ cup (30g) chopped raw or roasted hazelnuts or pecans

Freshly ground black pepper

- Heat 2 tablespoons (30 ml) of the dressing in a small frying pan over medium-low heat. Add the kale, radishes, and nuts. Cover and cook for about 5 minutes, stirring occasionally, until the kale has wilted.

- Remove from the heat and divide between 2 plates to serve. Top with freshly ground pepper and the remaining dressing.

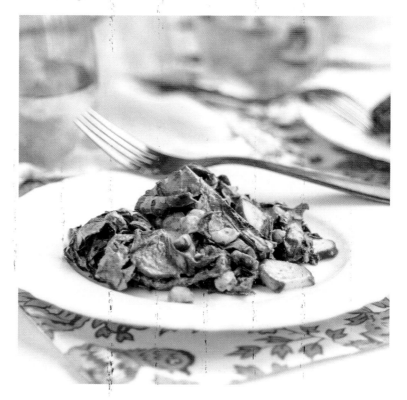

To store **Refrigerate in a tightly sealed container for up to 3 days.**

To reheat **Warm in a small frying pan over low heat for about 5 minutes, until the desired temperature is reached.**

NUTRITION INFORMATION: **238** calories | **22.9g** fat | **4g** protein | **6.7g** total carbs | **3.3g** net carbs

Portabella and Summer Squash Salad

This side salad is easy to throw together and pairs well with my keto Black Bean Burgers (page 144) or your favorite burger substitute. If you've got a little extra time to spend on meal prep, try marinating the mushrooms and squash in the dressing for about 15 minutes and then grilling them before assembling the salad.

 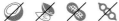

YIELD: 2 servings   PREP TIME: 5 minutes (not including time to make dressing)   COOK TIME: 5 minutes

2 tablespoons (30 ml) Greek Dressing (page 188)

²/₃ cup (100g) thinly sliced summer squash

2 large portabella mushrooms (about 6 inches/15 cm in diameter), gills and stems removed, sliced

2 cups (40g) baby arugula

2 tablespoons (15g) raw or roasted sunflower seeds

- Heat the dressing in a medium-sized frying pan over medium-low heat.

- Add the squash slices and mushrooms and cook for about 5 minutes, until they are tender.

- Divide the arugula between 2 bowls. Top each bowl with half of the cooked vegetables and a tablespoon of sunflower seeds.

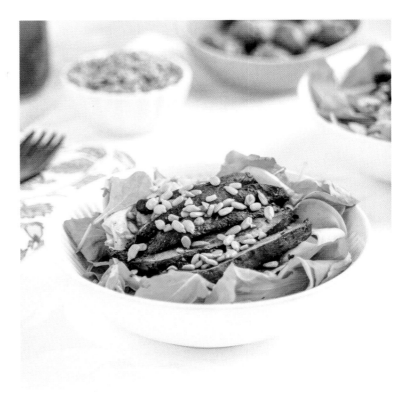

To store **Refrigerate in a tightly sealed container for up to 2 days.**

Variation WILTED GREENS SALAD WITH PORTABELLA AND SUMMER SQUASH. **Add the arugula to the pan with the mushrooms. Cover and cook for about 5 minutes, until the mushrooms and squash are cooked through and the arugula is wilted. Divide between 2 bowls and top with the sunflower seeds.**

NUTRITION INFORMATION: **169** calories | **14.2g** fat | **5.3g** protein | **10.9g** total carbs | **5.3g** net carbs

Green Keto Balance Bowl

Veggie bowls are a great way to use up extra greens and other assorted veg you have lying around. Typically, these bowls involve rice or grains, steamed or roasted veggies, and some nuts, seeds, and/or herbs. The keto version of this aesthetically pleasing meal replaces the rice with cauliflower rice but still follows the same formula—loads of fresh veggies arranged in a fun way. Does it need to be Instagram-worthy? Probably not, but where's the fun in that?

This particular bowl is my favorite combination of ingredients. It's got heaps of protein and a nice amount of fiber and is quite filling. You can customize this bowl to your own tastes by replacing any of the ingredients with your own favorite low-carb ones!

   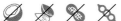

YIELD: 2 servings   PREP TIME: 10 minutes (not including time to cook vegetables or make dressing)

1 cup (150g) cooked Cauliflower Rice (page 178)

1 cup (190g) cooked spinach

1 cup (100g) bite-sized roasted broccoli florets

1 medium Hass avocado (7½ ounces/212g), sliced

½ cup (60g) raw pepitas (pumpkin seeds)

¼ cup (40g) hulled hemp seeds

2 tablespoons (20g) sesame seeds (black or white)

¼ cup (60 ml) Tahini Dressing (page 186)

FOR GARNISH (OPTIONAL):

Broccoli sprouts

Fresh cilantro leaves

Lime wedges

- Divide the cauliflower rice, spinach, broccoli, avocado, pepitas, and hemp seeds between 2 bowls. Top each bowl with 1 tablespoon (10 g) of sesame seeds and 2 tablespoons (30 ml) of the dressing.

- Garnish as desired.

To store Refrigerate the bowl ingredients separate from the dressing in a tightly sealed container for up to 3 days.

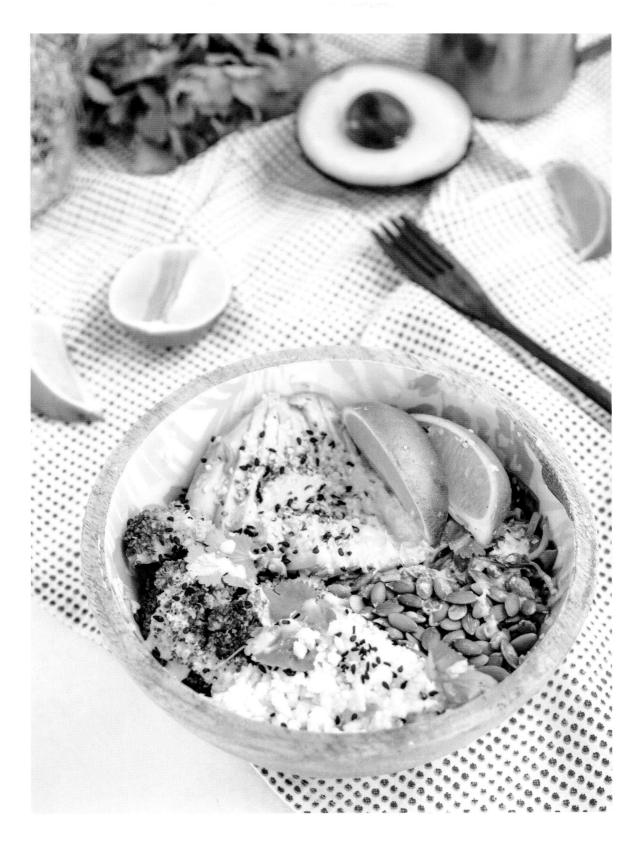

Taco Salad

I don't remember when I first discovered that you could use chopped walnuts in place of ground meat (after some soaking or heating, of course), but it was a total game-changer for me. Walnuts are my favorite meat replacement, tastewise. Although it does take some extra time, it's definitely worth soaking the walnuts in water for at least 30 minutes prior to using them in this recipe. I've tried to get away with cooking the nuts on the stovetop for a little bit longer, but they don't soften up quite as much.

YIELD: 2 servings   PREP TIME: 8 minutes, plus time to soak nuts (not including time to make mayo)   COOK TIME: 5 minutes

1 cup (120g) raw walnuts

¼ cup (60 ml) vegetable broth

1 teaspoon chili powder

1 teaspoon dried oregano leaves

½ teaspoon ground cumin

¼ teaspoon granulated garlic

¼ teaspoon paprika

¼ teaspoon salt

4 cups (120g) chopped lettuce or mixed baby greens

¼ cup (60 ml) salsa

¼ cup (60 ml) Tangy Avocado Mayo (page 183)

FOR GARNISH (OPTIONAL):

Fresh cilantro leaves

Lime juice

- To prepare the walnuts, either cover them with cold water and place in the fridge to soak overnight or cover with near-boiling water and soak for 30 minutes.

- To make the taco filling, drain the soaked walnuts, then transfer them to a blender or food processor and pulse until they have the texture of cooked ground beef.

- Place the chopped walnuts, broth, and seasonings in a small saucepan over medium heat, stir, and cook for about 5 minutes, until most of the broth has been absorbed. Remove from the heat and let cool for 5 minutes. The walnuts should have absorbed all of the liquid.

- Divide the lettuce between 2 serving bowls. Top each bowl with half of the taco filling, 2 tablespoons (30 ml) of salsa, and 2 tablespoons (30 ml) of mayo. Garnish with cilantro and a squeeze of lime juice, if desired.

To store: Refrigerate the components separately in tightly sealed containers for up to 3 days.

Notes: You can replace the spices with 1 tablespoon of your favorite taco seasoning. Be sure to check whether it contains salt before adding that in!

If you don't have any Tangy Avocado Mayo on hand, you can always replace it with guacamole or plain avocado slices.

NUTRITION INFORMATION: **505** calories | **47.9g** fat | **11.1g** protein | **15.6g** total carbs | **7.8g** net carbs

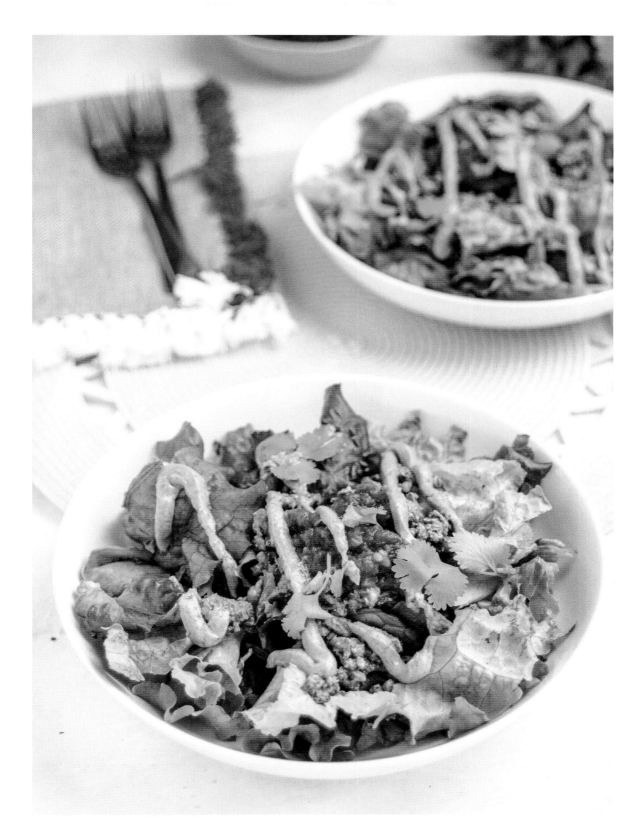

Greek Salad

Greek salads tend to be my go-to order at restaurants. They're pretty easy to veganize, and I've never been disappointed by a dish that features Kalamata olives! You can make this salad a meal by adding 4 ounces (112 grams) of baked or grilled tofu or tempeh or a serving of mock chicken.

  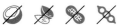

YIELD: 2 servings
PREP TIME: 5 minutes (not including time to make dressing)

3 lightly packed cups (90g) fresh baby spinach

½ cup (50g) sliced cucumbers

¼ cup (30g) halved cherry tomatoes

2 ounces (56g) pitted Kalamata olives

¼ cup (30g) raw or roasted sunflower seeds

¼ cup (60 ml) Greek Dressing (page 188)

Divide the spinach, cucumbers, tomatoes, and olives between 2 bowls and top each salad with half of the sunflower seeds and dressing.

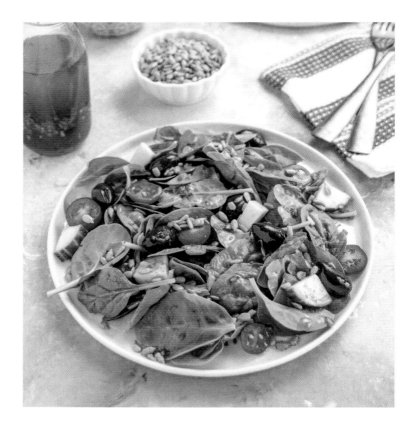

To store **Refrigerate without dressing for up to 3 days.**

NUTRITION INFORMATION: **328** calories | **32g** fat | **5.1g** protein | **7.2g** total carbs | **4.3g** net carbs

Garlic Ginger Slaw

This slaw has become such a staple at our family dinners that my sister-in-law had me write out the recipe and stick it on her fridge. The ingredients and method are simple, but this side dish packs some major flavor! While it's delicious anytime, I think it tastes best after it's left in the fridge for about an hour so that all the flavors can blend together.

YIELD: 4 servings   PREP TIME: 15 minutes

DRESSING:

1 tablespoon low-sodium tamari or coconut aminos

1 tablespoon toasted sesame oil

1 tablespoon unseasoned rice wine vinegar

½ teaspoon crushed garlic

½ teaspoon grated fresh ginger

2 cups (140g) thinly sliced red cabbage

2 cups (140g) thinly sliced green cabbage

¼ cup (30g) shredded carrots

¼ cup (20g) sliced scallions (green parts only)

2 tablespoons (20g) sesame seeds

- To make the dressing, whisk together the ingredients for the dressing in a small bowl and set aside.

- Put both types of cabbage, the carrots, scallions, and sesame seeds in a large salad bowl.

- Pour the dressing over the slaw mixture and toss well. If desired, chill in the fridge for an hour to let the flavors combine a bit before serving, or serve immediately.

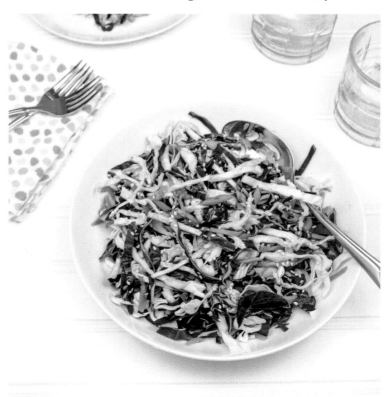

To store: *Refrigerate in a tightly sealed container for up to 5 days.*

Mediterranean Zucchini Salad

The first time I made this dish, I ate about half of it on the spot because it was so good. Within about ten minutes, my husband had come downstairs and finished the rest. I made another batch instantly so that we would have some in the fridge for later.

I often toss a serving of this salad with a big bowl of baby spinach and an additional ¼ cup (30g) of sunflower seeds to make it more filling.

YIELD: 4 servings   PREP TIME: 5 minutes (not including time to make noodles)

DRESSING:

1 tablespoon lemon juice

1 tablespoon extra-virgin olive oil

½ teaspoon crushed garlic

1 recipe Zucchini Noodles (page 179)

½ cup (83g) jarred lupini beans (packed in brine), drained

4 ounces (112g) pitted black olives, halved

¼ cup (30g) raw or roasted sunflower seeds

¼ cup (10g) sliced sun-dried tomatoes

- To make the dressing, whisk together the lemon juice, olive oil, and garlic in a medium-sized mixing bowl.

- Add the remaining ingredients to the bowl and toss with the dressing.

- Let the salad sit for about 15 minutes for the flavors to meld and the sun-dried tomatoes to rehydrate, then transfer to a serving dish.

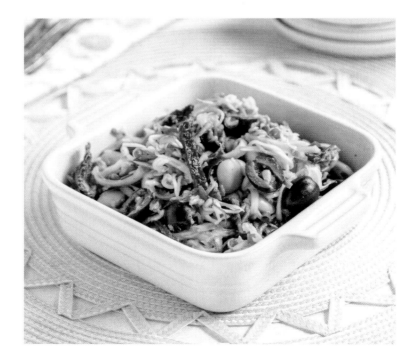

To store **Refrigerate in a tightly sealed container for up to 2 days.**

NUTRITION INFORMATION: **147** calories | **10.9g** fat | **6g** protein | **8.9g** total carbs | **5.8g** net carbs

Lemon Pesto Greens

I would happily eat the whole batch of these greens without batting an eye. In fact, that's usually what happens when I make them. I like to change up the greens I use to add interest and because different greens are available at different times of the year. While you can make this recipe with chard, collard, kale, mustard greens, or pretty much any other type of green, I highly recommend broccoli rabe (I used just the leaves here), which is higher in protein and lower in carbs than most other veggies.

   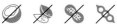

YIELD: 4 servings   PREP TIME: 5 minutes (not including time to make pesto)   COOK TIME: 10 minutes

¹/₃ cup (80 ml) Easy Vegan Pesto (page 189)

Grated zest and juice of 1 lemon

4 cups (160g) chopped broccoli rabe or other green(s) of choice

¼ teaspoon salt

- Heat the pesto with the lemon juice and zest in a large frying pan over medium heat.

- Add the chopped greens and sprinkle with the salt. Cover and cook for 5 minutes, until the greens have wilted to about half their original volume.

- Stir to coat the greens in the pesto. Cover and cook for another 5 to 10 minutes, until the leaves and stems are tender.

- Transfer to a serving dish to enjoy.

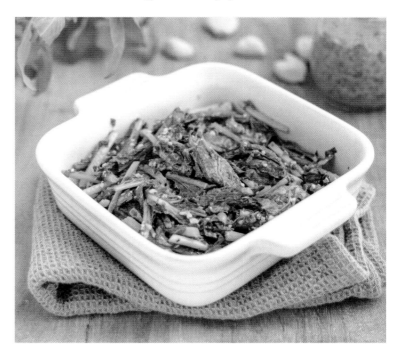

To store Refrigerate in a tightly sealed container for up to 3 days.

To reheat Place in a small frying pan over low heat for about 5 minutes, until the desired temperature is reached.

Cucumber Salad

I love eating this cucumber salad at summer cookouts. It's refreshing yet filling, and it readily takes the place of potato salad without trying to be potato salad. While you can serve this salad immediately after assembling it, I think the overall taste improves when the flavors have at least an hour to mingle in the fridge.

   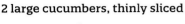

YIELD: 4 servings   PREP TIME: 10 minutes, plus time to chill (not including time to make sour cream)

2 large cucumbers, thinly sliced

1 teaspoon salt

½ cup (120 ml) Quick Hemp Seed Sour Cream (page 185)

½ cup (10g) chopped fresh dill leaves

¼ teaspoon cracked black pepper

Paprika, for sprinkling

- In a large mixing bowl, toss the cucumber slices with the salt. Let sit in the refrigerator for 30 minutes. The cucumbers will release some of their liquid.

- After 30 minutes, pour the excess liquid out of the bowl and place the cucumber slices in the center of a clean dish towel. Using the towel, squeeze out the excess moisture from the cucumbers—they should look darker green and somewhat translucent.

- Return the cucumber slices to the empty mixing bowl and stir in the sour cream, dill, and pepper. Mix until everything is evenly distributed.

- Cover and place in the refrigerator to chill for 1 hour to let the flavors combine.

- To serve, divide the salad among 4 plates and sprinkle a pinch of paprika over each serving.

To store **Refrigerate in a tightly sealed container for up to 2 days.**

NUTRITION INFORMATION: **161** calories | **13.4g** fat | **6.1g** protein | **7.3g** total carbs | **4.7g** net carbs

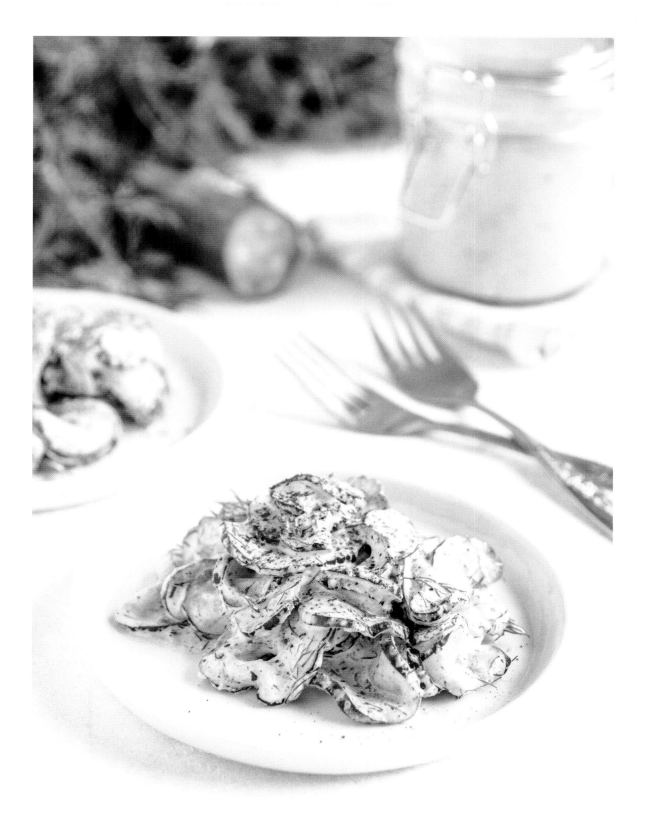

Chili Tamari Tofu

Loaded with protein and low in carbs, this spicy tofu is sure to give any meal a little kick. I usually add a serving (or two!) to slaws, salads, and noodle dishes if I haven't already covered them in hemp seeds.

1 (14-ounce/397-g) block extra-firm tofu

2 tablespoons (30 ml) low-sodium tamari or coconut aminos

1 tablespoon extra-virgin olive oil

1 tablespoon chili paste or Sriracha sauce

YIELD: 4 servings PREP TIME: 10 minutes COOK TIME: 25 minutes

- Preheat the oven to 350°F (177°C) and line a rimmed baking sheet with parchment paper or a silicone baking mat.

- Drain the tofu and press out any excess liquid.

- Cut the tofu in half lengthwise, then cut each half into ½-inch (1.25-cm) thick slices.

- In a small dish, whisk together the tamari, olive oil, and chili paste. Dip each piece of tofu in the tamari mixture and place on the baking sheet. Brush or pour the remainder of the sauce onto the tofu pieces.

- Bake for 25 minutes, until crispy around the edges, flipping the tofu over halfway through baking. Enjoy warm.

To store **Refrigerate in a tightly sealed container for up to 4 days.**

To reheat **Place in a preheated 300°F (150°C) oven for about 5 minutes, until warmed through.**

NUTRITION INFORMATION: **128** calories | **8.1g** fat | **11.2g** protein | **4g** total carbs | **2.6g** net carbs

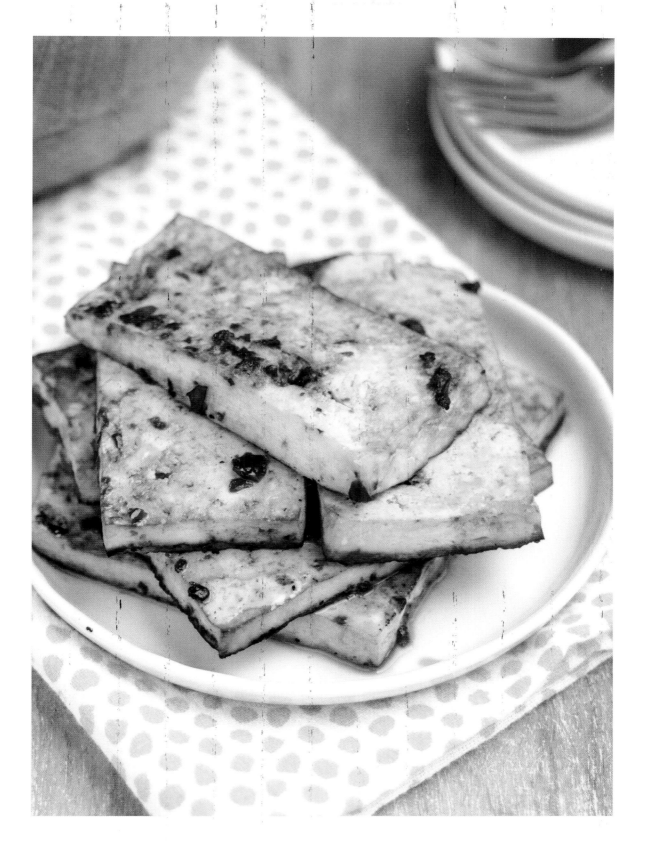

Tangy Brussels Sprouts with Mushrooms & Walnuts

Brussels sprouts, mushrooms, and walnuts just seem like a natural combination to me, and I eat them together constantly. While they're so delicious on their own that they really don't need much else, roasting B-sprouts (as my best friend calls them) in mustard dressing is an easy way to add loads of flavor.

YIELD: 4 servings   PREP TIME: 5 minutes (not including time to make vinaigrette)   COOK TIME: 30 minutes

2 cups (240g) trimmed and halved Brussels sprouts

2 cups (192g) sliced cremini mushrooms

¼ cup (30g) coarsely chopped raw walnuts

¼ cup (60 ml) Easy Mustard Vinaigrette (page 184)

- Preheat the oven to 375°F (190°C) and line a rimmed baking sheet with parchment paper.

- In a large mixing bowl, toss the Brussels sprouts, mushrooms, and walnuts in the dressing until completely coated. Spread in a single layer on the lined baking sheet.

- Bake for 25 to 30 minutes, until the Brussels sprouts turn golden brown and are tender enough to easily pierce with a knife.

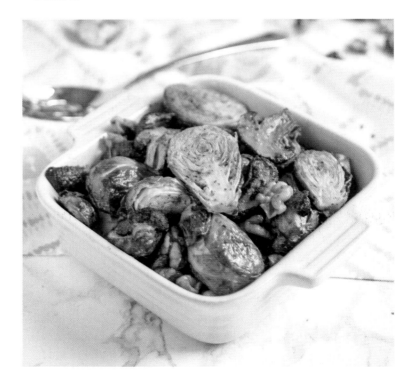

To store Refrigerate in a tightly sealed container for up to 3 days.

To reheat Place in a small frying pan over low heat for about 5 minutes, until the desired temperature is reached.

Crispy Broccoli Bites

Broccoli is one of my favorite vegetables. I usually just roast or steam it plain and dig in, but sometimes I like to dress it up a bit. These crispy broccoli bites are so tasty that my husband actually requests I make an entire separate batch just for him. I've included reheating instructions just in case, but I can't remember the last time I made a batch that lasted long enough to be stored in the refrigerator. It's well worth saving up your carbs for!

YIELD: 4 servings   PREP TIME: 5 minutes   COOK TIME: 30 minutes

¼ cup (64g) tahini, room temperature

2 tablespoons (30 ml) low-sodium tamari or coconut aminos

2 tablespoons (30 ml) extra-virgin olive oil

2 tablespoons (30 ml) water

2 tablespoons (14g) ground flax seeds

1 teaspoon crushed garlic

1 teaspoon grated fresh ginger

3 cups (210g) broccoli florets

- Preheat the oven to 350°F (177°C) and line a rimmed baking sheet with parchment paper.
- Place all the ingredients except the broccoli in a medium-sized mixing bowl and mix until smooth.
- Add the broccoli and stir until the florets are coated with the tahini mixture.
- Spread the florets in a single layer on the lined baking sheet and bake for 30 minutes, until crispy.

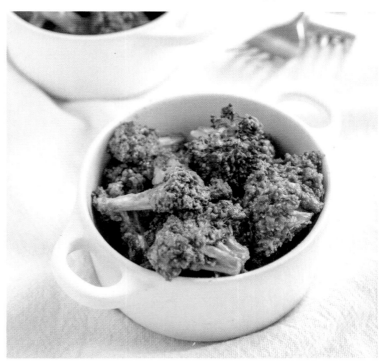

To store Refrigerate in a tightly sealed container for up to 3 days.

To reheat Place in a preheated 300°F (150°C) oven for about 5 minutes, until warmed through.

Sweet Chili Roasted Radishes

Right off the bat, I want to make sure something is clear—I'm not going to try to pass these off as some sort of roasted potato substitute. They're radishes, and they taste like radishes. They also taste absolutely delicious, though to be fair, I think anything covered in sweet chili sauce tastes pretty darn good.

YIELD: 4 servings   PREP TIME: 10 minutes   COOK TIME: 30 minutes

2 tablespoons (30 ml) low-sodium tamari or coconut aminos

2 tablespoons (30 ml) extra-virgin olive oil

2 teaspoons chili paste or Sriracha sauce

2 teaspoons granulated sweetener

1 pound (454g) radishes

2 tablespoons (20g) sesame seeds

2 scallions (green parts only), sliced

• Preheat the oven to 375°F (190°C) and line a rimmed baking sheet with parchment paper.

• In a small bowl, whisk together the tamari, olive oil, chili paste, and sweetener.

• Trim and quarter the radishes and put them in a medium-sized mixing bowl. Pour the tamari mixture over the radishes and toss to coat.

• Spread the radishes on the lined baking sheet and pour any remaining sauce from the bowl over them.

• Bake for 30 minutes, until tender. Toss with the sesame seeds and sliced scallions. Transfer to a serving dish or divide among 4 plates to serve.

To store **Refrigerate in a tightly sealed container for up to 3 days.**

To reheat **Spread on a rimmed baking sheet lined with parchment paper and heat in a preheated 300°F (150°C) oven for about 5 minutes, until warmed through.**

Note **If you find that sugar alcohols upset your stomach, you can try using ⅛ teaspoon of liquid stevia instead of the granulated sweetener.**

NUTRITION INFORMATION: **112** calories | **9.8g** fat | **2.5g** protein | **4.9g** total carbs | **2.2g** net carbs

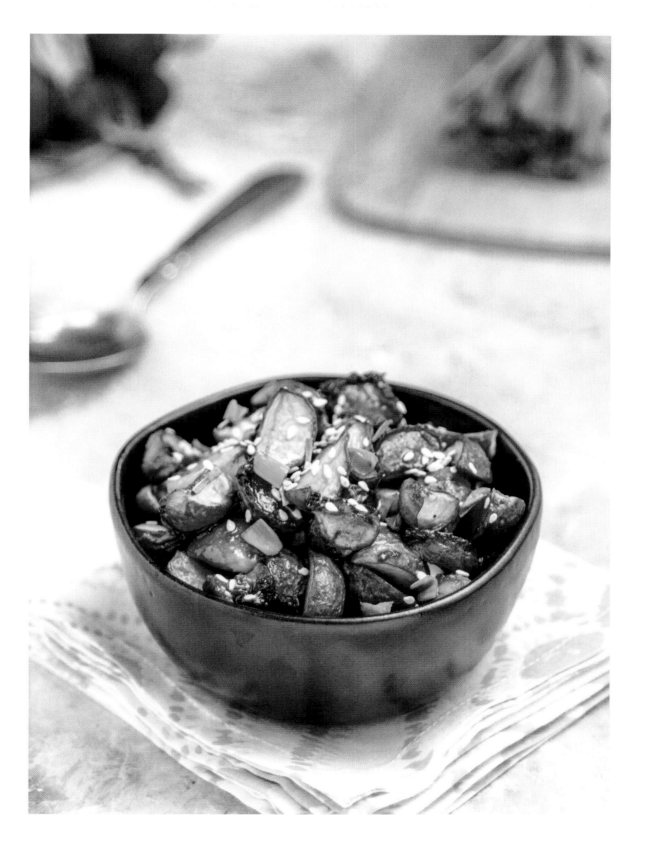

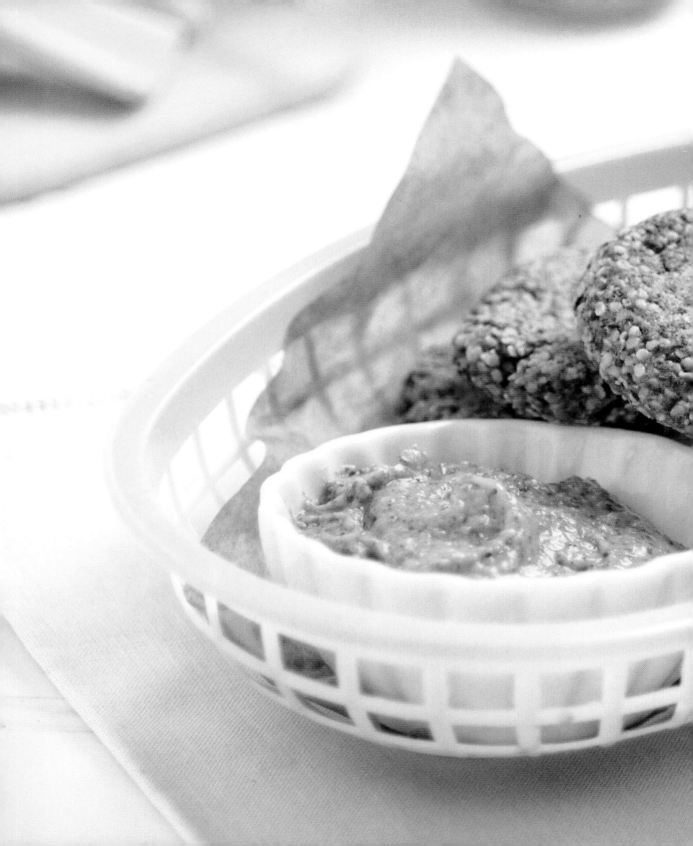

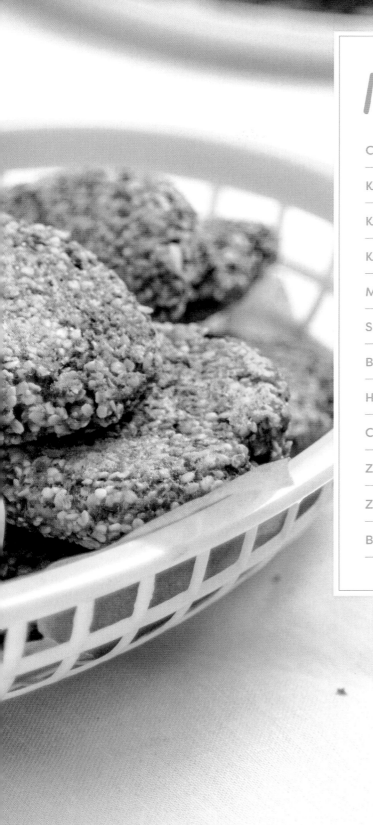

Main Courses

Cabbage Rolls

No dish reminds me more of my childhood than cabbage rolls. Every time there was a family gathering, my Aunt Lyn would make trays and trays of these—called *gołąbki* (go-WUMP-ki) in Polish—and I don't recall there being any leftovers. This is a keto-fied and vegan version of my aunt's dish, and every time I make it, I think of her.

YIELD: 4 rolls (1 per serving)   PREP TIME: 20 minutes, plus time to soak nuts   COOK TIME: 50 minutes

1 cup (120g) raw walnuts

4 large green cabbage leaves (see Note)

1 tablespoon extra-virgin olive oil

2 tablespoons (25g) finely chopped onions

½ teaspoon salt

¼ teaspoon ground black pepper

¼ teaspoon paprika

¾ cup (85g) Cauliflower Rice (page 178), uncooked

1 tablespoon dried parsley leaves

1 Flax Egg (page 182)

½ cup (120 ml) low-sugar tomato sauce

- To prepare the walnuts, place them in a small dish and either cover with cold water and let soak in the fridge overnight or cover with near-boiling water and let soak for 30 minutes.

- Preheat the oven to 350°F (177°C).

- Pour enough water into a large pot to come ½ inch (1.25 cm) up the sides. Cover and bring to a simmer. Add the cabbage leaves, cover, and steam until the leaves are soft and pliable, about 5 minutes.

- Meanwhile, heat the olive oil in a frying pan over medium-low heat. Add the onions, salt, pepper, and paprika and cook, stirring frequently, until the onions begin to sweat and turn translucent. Add the cauliflower, stir to combine, and turn the heat down to low. Continue cooking until the rice is soft, about 10 minutes.

- When the cabbage is done, remove the leaves from the pot, drain, and let cool.

- Drain the soaked walnuts and put them in a blender or food processor. Pulse until they have the consistency of cooked ground beef. Add the ground walnuts, parsley, and flax egg to the frying pan with the rice and stir to combine. Turn off the heat.

- Once the cabbage leaves are cool enough to handle, carefully cut out the large vein that runs down the middle of each leaf. Finely chop the veins and stir them into the walnuts and cauliflower.

Note Remove 4 large cabbage leaves from a head of cabbage by coring the head, then carefully peeling the leaves away. I find it helpful to start at the thick stem of each leaf and work outward.

To store Refrigerate in a tightly sealed container for up to 5 days.

To reheat Place in a preheated 300°F (150°C) oven for 10 minutes, until warmed through.

NUTRITION INFORMATION: **254** calories | **23.6g** fat | **6.1g** protein | **9.1g** total carbs | **5.3g** net carbs

- Spread a cabbage leaf out flat on a clean work surface and spoon one-quarter of the walnut mixture in a line across the top of the leaf, making sure to leave at least ½ inch of space for wrapping. Starting at the ends, fold the edges of the leaf around the filling, then wrap the rest of the leaf around the filling. Lay the roll seam side down in a 1½-quart (1.5-L) casserole dish. Repeat with the remaining leaves and filling, making a total of 4 rolls.

- Spoon the tomato sauce over the rolls and bake for 30 minutes, until the sauce around the edges begins to darken and bubble.

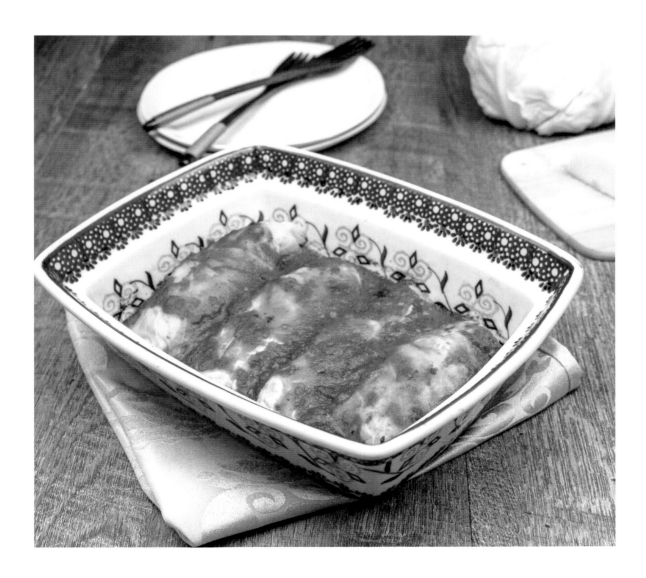

Kelp Noodle Pad Thai

This is one of those little treats that I like to make for myself whenever I'm craving takeout. Not only do the kelp noodles provide more than 50 percent of the daily recommended intake for iodine, but they also contain more than 20 percent of the DRI for calcium. To make this a meal and increase the protein, add one serving of Chili Tamari Tofu (page 126) to each serving of pad Thai.

YIELD: 2 servings
PREP TIME: 10 minutes, plus time to soften noodles in dressing (optional)

1 (12-ounce/340-g) package kelp noodles, drained

DRESSING:

2 tablespoons (32g) unsweetened creamy almond butter

1 tablespoon low-sodium tamari or coconut aminos

1 tablespoon toasted sesame oil

1 tablespoon water

1 clove garlic, crushed to a paste

2 tablespoons (20g) sesame seeds

¼ cup (30g) raw pepitas (pumpkin seeds)

FOR GARNISH:

1 tablespoon shredded carrots

2 scallions (green parts only), sliced

2 teaspoons sesame seeds

- Put the kelp noodles in a colander. Rinse thoroughly, then set aside to drain.

- In a mixing bowl, whisk together the ingredients for the dressing.

- Pat the noodles dry and add them to the bowl with the dressing. Toss the noodles in the dressing and let sit for 20 minutes so that the dressing soaks into the noodles and softens them. For a crunchier dish, skip this resting period.

- Stir the pepitas into the noodles, then divide the noodles between 2 plates or bowls. Garnish with the carrots, scallions, and sesame seeds.

To store **Refrigerate in a tightly sealed container for up to 2 days.**

NUTRITION INFORMATION: **338** calories | **30.2g** fat | **10.6g** protein | **14g** total carbs | **7.9g** net carbs

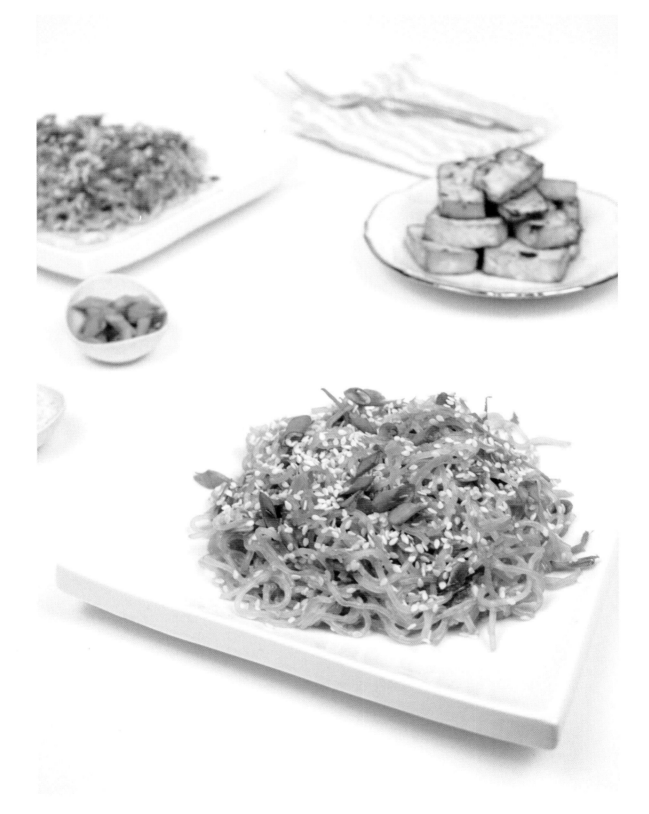

Keto Pot Pie

Warm, rich, and filling, this pot pie is the perfect dish to eat on a cold day.

I like to make my own nut flours to save a little money. You can easily make your own nut flours by simply grinding whole nuts in a food processor or high-powered blender. See page 176 for detailed instructions on how to make and store nut flours.

YIELD: 4 servings   PREP TIME: 20 minutes   COOK TIME: 30 minutes

CRUST:

1 cup (112g) finely ground blanched almond flour

1 tablespoon (5g) psyllium husks

Pinch of salt

2 tablespoons (30 ml) water

FILLING:

½ cup (80g) hulled hemp seeds

½ cup (80g) jarred lupini beans (packed in brine), drained

¾ cup (180 ml) vegetable broth

2 tablespoons (30 ml) extra-virgin olive oil

¼ cup (20g) nutritional yeast

1 tablespoon Savory Herb Blend (page 175) or poultry herb seasoning of choice

1 lightly packed cup (30g) chopped fresh spinach

1 cup (90g) chopped broccoli florets, fresh or frozen, thawed if frozen

½ cup (70g) cubed canned young jackfruit (packed in brine), drained and chopped

- Preheat the oven to 350°F (177°C). Have on hand a 1- to 1½-quart (1- to 1.5-L) casserole dish.

- To make the crust, whisk together the almond flour, psyllium husks, and salt. Stir in the water until a dough forms. Knead until uniform, then roll out between 2 sheets of wax or parchment paper until it is slightly larger than the top of the casserole dish you are using.

- To make the sauce for the filling, put the hemp seeds, lupini beans, broth, and olive oil in a high-powered blender or food processor and process until creamy and smooth, about 2 minutes. If the mixture still feels a little gritty after 2 minutes, keep blending!

- Turn off the blender and add the nutritional yeast and herb seasoning. Pulse a few times to mix in the herbs without pulverizing them completely.

- Put the spinach, broccoli, and jackfruit in a large mixing bowl. Pour the sauce from the blender over the vegetables, then stir to combine. Scoop the filling into the casserole dish.

- Peel the top sheet of wax paper off the rolled-out crust and carefully flip the crust over the casserole dish to cover. Peel back the remaining sheet of paper and press and crimp the crust all around the edge of the dish to seal it. If any crust is hanging over the side of the dish, remove it and press it into any visible cracks. Cut four 1-inch (2.5-cm) slits in the top of the crust so that steam can escape.

- Bake the pot pie until the crust is uniform in color and firm to the touch, 25 minutes if using a 1.5-quart (1.5-L) casserole dish or 30 minutes if using a 1-quart (1-L) dish. Remove from the oven and let cool for 20 minutes before serving.

To store: Cover and refrigerate for up to 4 days.

To reheat: Place in a preheated 300°F (150°C) oven for 15 minutes, until warmed through.

Tip: While the crust is easy to work with, it is imperative that you roll it out between sheets of wax or parchment paper. Without the paper, it will stick to the counter and your rolling pin.

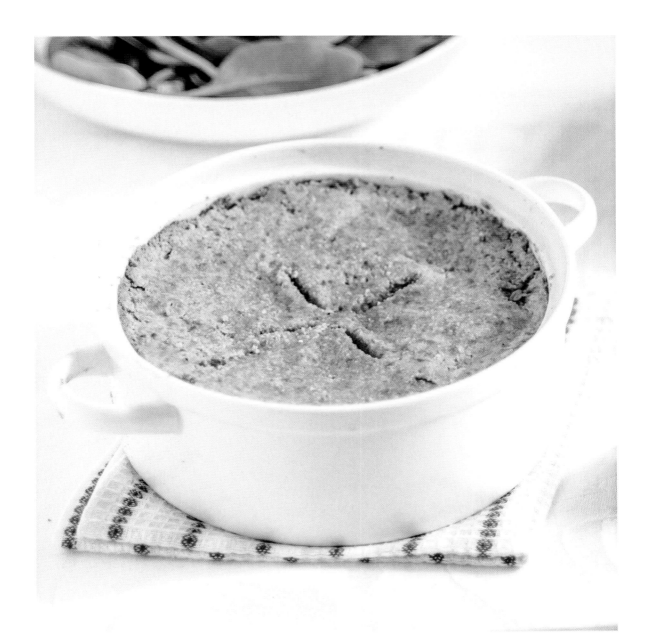

Korean BBQ Tacos

The inspiration for these tacos came from a free recipe card for Korean BBQ beef tacos from one of those meal prep box subscriptions. After some (pretty major) tweaking and a lot of trial and error, one of my favorite dinner recipes was born. Normally I struggle to find the patience to soak nuts for recipes, but this one is worth it. If you don't already have a batch of flax tortillas on hand, I recommend making them when the nuts are nearly done soaking.

  YIELD: 6 small tacos (2 per serving)   PREP TIME: 15 minutes, plus time to soak nuts (not including time to make tortillas or mayo)   COOK TIME: 5 minutes

FILLING:

1 cup (120g) raw walnuts

SAUCE:

¼ cup (60 ml) low-sodium tamari or coconut aminos

1 tablespoon toasted sesame oil

1 teaspoon chili paste or Sriracha sauce

1 teaspoon grated fresh ginger

2 cloves garlic, minced

A few drops of liquid stevia (optional)

1 recipe Flax Tortillas (page 180), or 6 small low-carb tortillas of choice

FOR GARNISH:

¼ heaping cup (20g) thinly sliced red cabbage

3 tablespoons (15g) sliced scallions (green parts only)

1 teaspoon sesame seeds

3 tablespoons (45 ml) Tangy Avocado Mayo (page 183)

- To prepare the walnuts, place them in a small dish and either cover with cold water and let soak in the fridge overnight or cover with near-boiling water and let soak for 30 minutes.

- To make the filling, drain the soaked walnuts, then place them in a blender or food processor and pulse until they have the consistency of cooked ground beef.

- In a small mixing bowl, whisk together the ingredients for the sauce.

- Put the processed walnuts in a large frying pan over medium-low heat and pour the sauce on top. Cook for about 5 minutes, moving the walnuts around in the pan every minute or so, until the sauce is mostly absorbed.

- To assemble the tacos, place about ¼ cup (30g) of the walnut filling in each tortilla, then garnish evenly with the cabbage, scallions, sesame seeds, and avocado mayo.

To store: Refrigerate the ingredients separately for up to 3 days. The leftovers are best eaten cold.

NUTRITION INFORMATION: **560** calories | **50.8g** fat | **15.2g** protein | **19.5g** total carbs | **5.3g** net carbs

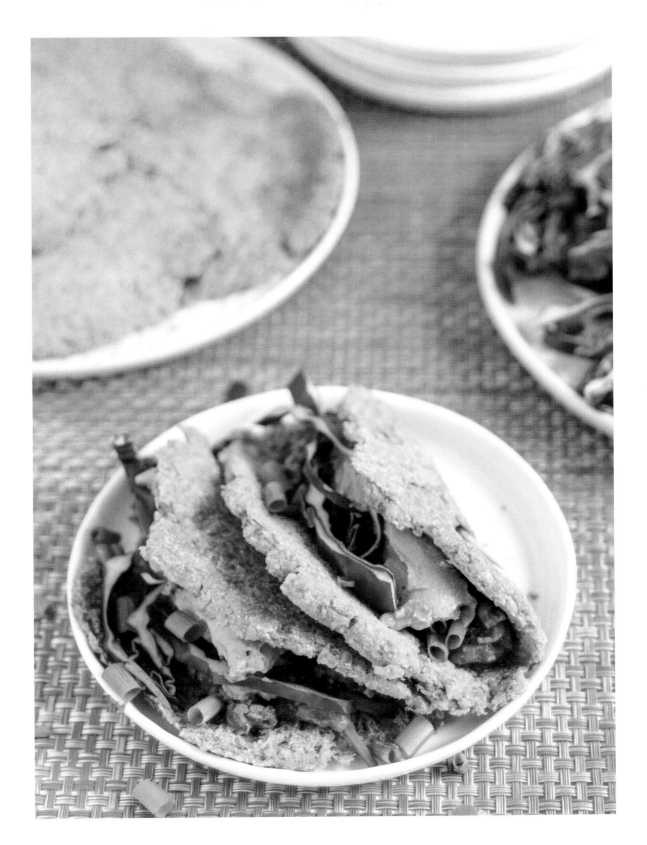

Meal Prep Chili

The most common recipe request I get is for big-batch slow cooker dinners. I get it—sometimes you just want to make one thing to bring to lunch for work during the week. It's one less thing to think about. This simple and flavorful chili is my favorite thing to batch cook for the week. I usually serve it over chopped spinach, but it works just as well over a bowl of cauliflower rice.

YIELD: 6 servings   PREP TIME: 10 minutes
COOK TIME: 30 minutes to 6 hours

2 (15-ounce/425-g) cans black soybeans, drained and rinsed

2 cups (200g) sliced celery

1 cup (240 ml) low-sugar tomato sauce

1 cup (240 ml) vegetable broth

1 cup (120g) chopped raw walnuts

2 teaspoons crushed garlic

2 tablespoons (10g) chili powder

1 teaspoon granulated onion

FOR SERVING:

6 lightly packed cups (180g) chopped fresh spinach

2 scallions (green parts only), sliced

- To make in a slow cooker: Place all the chili ingredients in a slow cooker. Cover and cook for 6 hours on low or about 3 hours on high, until the celery is tender and the walnuts have softened.

- To make on the stovetop: Heat all the chili ingredients in a medium-sized pot or Dutch oven over medium heat, covered, for about 30 minutes, until the celery is tender and the walnuts have softened.

- Place 1 cup of chopped spinach in each bowl and top with the chili. Garnish with sliced scallions.

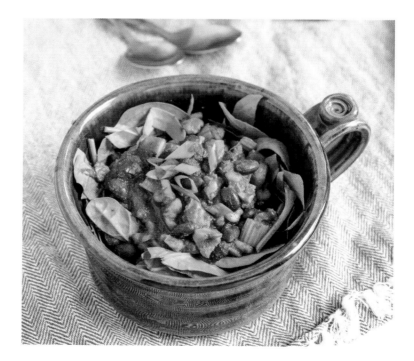

To store: Refrigerate the chili and spinach separately in tightly sealed containers. The chili will keep for up to a week.

To reheat: Microwave individual portions until heated through.

NUTRITION INFORMATION: **305** calories | **21.5g** fat | **16.8g** protein | **16.8g** total carbs | **5.1g** net carbs

Smashed Bean Sandwiches

So, this filling is definitely more "chopped in a food processor" than "smashed," but "smashed" sounds more fun, so that's what we're going with. These sandwiches are super filling and serve up quite a bit of protein.

Sometimes when I'm feeling lazy and don't want to bother making my own mayo (or cleaning the blender), I'll buy some vegan chipotle mayo and use that instead of the Tangy Avocado Mayo. I would definitely recommend it.

YIELD: 4 sandwiches (1 per serving)
PREP TIME: 10 minutes (not including time to make mayo or bread)

1 cup (166g) jarred lupini beans (packed in brine), drained

½ cup (50g) sliced celery

½ cup (120 ml) Tangy Avocado Mayo (page 183) or vegan mayo of choice

2 tablespoons (30 ml) prepared yellow mustard

8 thin slices Seed Bread (page 74)

OPTIONAL TOPPINGS:

Pickles

Lettuce

- Put the beans and celery in a blender or food processor and pulse about 10 times, until nicely chopped.

- Transfer the beans and celery to a small mixing bowl and add the mayo and mustard. Stir until everything is thoroughly combined.

- To make each sandwich, place one-fourth of the bean mixture on a slice of bread, then top with pickles and lettuce (if desired) and another slice of bread.

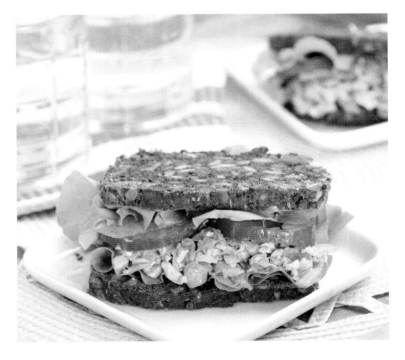

To store Refrigerate the smashed bean mixture, bread, and toppings separately. The bean mixture will keep for up to 1 day.

Black Bean Burgers

While there are plenty of burger substitutes out there, it's nice to be able to make your own low-carb version in a pinch. My favorite way to top these burgers is with sauerkraut, pickles, and mustard. Instead of a bun, I often opt to use a few lettuce leaves as a sort of wrap.

YIELD: 4 burgers (1 per serving)
PREP TIME: 5 minutes   COOK TIME: 45 minutes

1 (15-ounce/425-g) can unsalted black soybeans, drained and rinsed

¼ cup (40g) chia seeds, ground

1 teaspoon granulated garlic

1 tablespoon dehydrated onion flakes

3 tablespoons (45 ml) prepared yellow mustard

¼ teaspoon salt

Lettuce leaves, for serving

OPTIONAL TOPPINGS:

Pickle slices

Sauerkraut

Whole-grain mustard

- Preheat the oven to 350°F (177°C) and line a rimmed baking sheet with parchment paper.

- Using a blender or food processor, process all the burger ingredients until well combined. If some larger pieces of bean remain, that is fine!

- Form the mixture into 4 patties, about 3 inches (7.5 cm) in diameter and ½ inch (1.25 cm) thick, and place on the lined baking sheet.

- Bake for 45 minutes, flipping the burgers over halfway through the baking time. When done, they will be firm to the touch.

- Serve on lettuce leaves, topped as desired.

To store Refrigerate for up to 3 days or freeze, tightly wrapped, for up to a month.

To reheat Place in a preheated 300°F (150°C) oven for 5 minutes or until warmed through.

Variation SPICY BLACK BEAN BURGERS. *Replace the prepared yellow mustard with ¼ cup (60 ml) of salsa and add 1 tablespoon of chili powder to the bean mixture.*

NUTRITION INFORMATION (without toppings): **148** calories | **7.8g** fat | **10.4g** protein | **11.7g** total carbs | **1.2g** net carbs

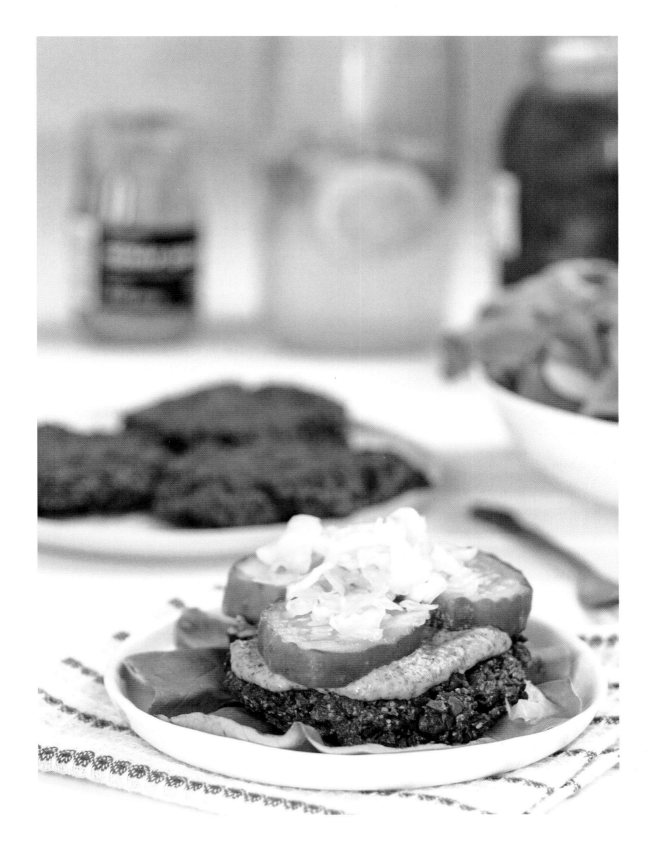

Hemp Seed Nuggets

You know when you have a ridiculous idea that comes out of nowhere? That's how these nuggets started. While browsing the mock meats at the grocery store and lamenting the lack of any sort of vegan nugget that is gluten-free and low-carb, I realized that this was one of those things I was going to have to make myself. After quite a bit of trial and error, these bad boys emerged from the oven, full of protein, omega-3 fatty acids, and deliciousness.

My favorite dipping sauce for these nuggets is whole-grain mustard, but they are also quite tasty with a vegan ranch dressing or my Tahini Dressing (page 186).

 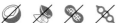

YIELD: 9 nuggets (3 per serving)
PREP TIME: 10 minutes   COOK TIME: 20 minutes

¾ cup (120g) hulled hemp seeds

½ cup (120 ml) vegetable broth

2 tablespoons (10g) nutritional yeast

1 tablespoon Savory Herb Blend (page 175) or poultry herb seasoning of choice

¼ teaspoon salt

¼ teaspoon ground black pepper

2 tablespoons (10g) psyllium husks

2 tablespoons (14g) unflavored pea protein powder or other unflavored vegan protein powder of choice

- Preheat the oven to 350°F (177°C) and line a rimmed baking sheet with parchment paper.

- In a blender or food processor, blend the hemp seeds, broth, nutritional yeast, herb blend, salt, and pepper. Transfer the mixture to a small bowl and stir in the psyllium husks and protein powder until the ingredients are thoroughly combined and a sticky dough forms.

- Using wet hands, shape the dough into 9 nuggets, about 2 tablespoons (30g) each, and place on the baking sheet.

- Bake for 20 minutes, flipping the nuggets over halfway through the baking time, until they are firm to the touch and slightly golden on the top and bottom.

To store Refrigerate for up to 3 days or freeze, tightly wrapped, for up to a month.

To reheat Place in a preheated 300°F (150°C) oven for 5 minutes or until warmed through.

Tip Wetting your hands before shaping the nuggets prevents the dough from sticking.

NUTRITION INFORMATION: **276** calories | **20.2g** fat | **19.5g** protein | **8.8g** total carbs | **3.4g** net carbs

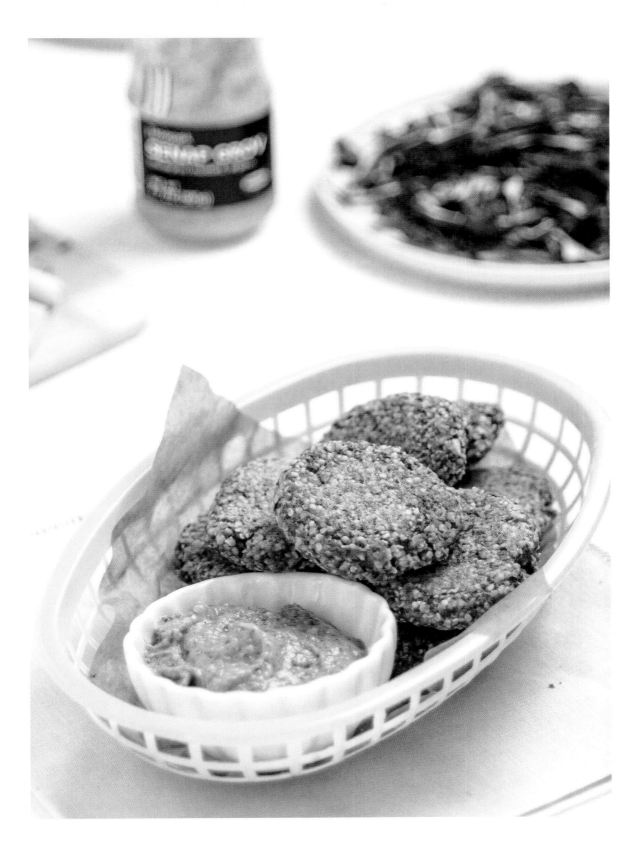

Cauliflower Bake

While "Cauliflower Bake" sounds really boring, this recipe is actually one of the most frequently made in my household. It's pretty easy to throw together and packs a ton of protein. If you get bored of cauliflower and don't mind the few extra carbs, I highly recommend making this with broccoli sometime, too.

YIELD: 4 servings   PREP TIME: 5 minutes (not including time to make sauce)
COOK TIME: 35 minutes

1 recipe Creamy Hemp Sauce (page 190)

6 cups (600g) cauliflower florets

½ cup (60g) raw pepitas (pumpkin seeds)

Ground black pepper

2 scallions (green parts only), sliced

- Preheat the oven to 375°F (190°C) and grease a 13 by 9-inch (33 by 23-cm) baking dish.

- In large mixing bowl, mix together the sauce, cauliflower florets, and pepitas. Transfer the mixture to the greased baking dish and season with pepper.

- Bake for 35 minutes, until the cauliflower is tender and the cauliflower is just starting to turn golden brown on top.

- Remove from the oven and top with the sliced scallions before serving.

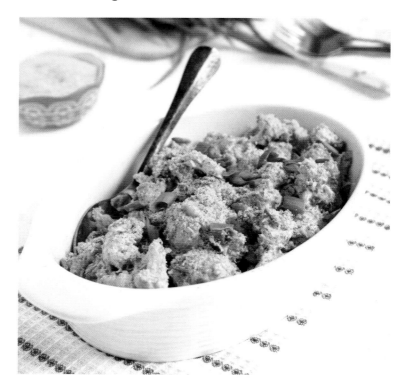

To store: Refrigerate in a tightly sealed container for up to 3 days or freeze for up to a month.

To reheat: Place in a preheated 300°F (150°C) oven for 10 to 15 minutes (or 25 to 30 minutes if frozen), until warmed through.

NUTRITION INFORMATION: **422** calories | **26g** fat | **30.5g** protein | **20g** total carbs | **7g** net carbs

Zucchini Bolognese

You know those nights when you're too tired to spend more than 15 minutes making dinner? This basic vegan keto version of spaghetti Bolognese is just the meal for those times.

2 tablespoons (30 ml) extra-virgin olive oil

1 (8-ounce/226-g) package tempeh

²/₃ cup (160 ml) low-sugar tomato sauce

1 recipe Zucchini Noodles (page 179), cooked

2 tablespoons (14g) Faux Parm Sprinkles (page 191)

Freshly ground black pepper

Thinly sliced fresh basil leaves, for garnish (optional)

YIELD: 2 servings   PREP TIME: 5 minutes (not including time to make noodles or sprinkles)   COOK TIME: 5 minutes

- Heat the olive oil in a medium-sized frying pan with a lid over medium heat. Using your hands, crumble the tempeh into the pan. Add the tomato sauce and stir.

- Cover and cook for about 5 minutes, until the tempeh is heated through. Remove the pan from the heat.

- Divide the zucchini noodles between 2 bowls and top each pile of noodles with half of the tempeh and sauce mixture. Top each dish with 1 tablespoon of Faux Parm Sprinkles and freshly ground pepper. Garnish with fresh basil, if desired.

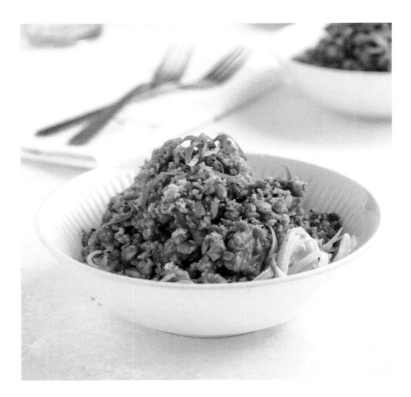

To store Refrigerate in a tightly sealed container for up to 2 days.

To reheat Warm in a medium-sized frying pan over medium-low heat, covered, for 5 minutes or until heated through.

NUTRITION INFORMATION: **455** calories | **35g** fat | **26.2g** protein | **15.8g** total carbs | **9.9g** net carbs

Zucchini Alfredo

This quick and easy meal is loaded with fiber, omega-3 fatty acids, protein, and (most importantly) flavor. I like to top it with Faux Parm Sprinkles or nutritional yeast for added B vitamins and even more protein.

  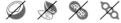

YIELD: 1 serving   PREP TIME: 2 minutes (not including time to make noodles, sauce, or sprinkles)   COOK TIME: 5 minutes

1½ cups (150g) raw Zucchini Noodles (page 179)

⅓ cup (80 ml) Creamy Hemp Sauce (page 190)

1 lightly packed cup (30g) chopped fresh spinach

SUGGESTED TOPPINGS:

1 tablespoon Faux Parm Sprinkles (page 191) or nutritional yeast

Freshly ground black pepper

Chopped fresh basil or parsley

Place the noodles, sauce, and spinach in a medium-sized saucepan over medium-low heat and stir until the noodles and spinach are coated in the sauce. Cover and cook for about 5 minutes, until the noodles are tender and the sauce is heated through. Place in a serving bowl and top as desired.

Variation RAW ZUCCHINI & SPINACH ALFREDO.
Stir together all the ingredients in a medium-sized mixing bowl, then transfer to a serving bowl or plate to serve. Top as desired.

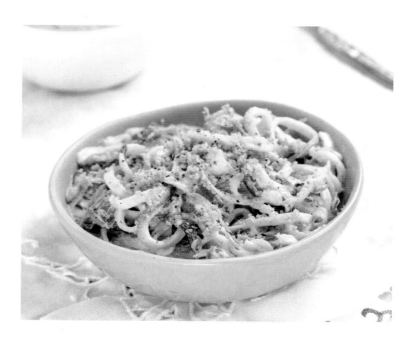

To store *Refrigerate in a tightly sealed container for up to 2 days.*

To reheat *Eat cold, or warm in a medium-sized frying pan over medium heat for about 5 minutes, until heated through.*

Buffalo Jackfruit Tacos

For many of the recipes in this book (and that I make for myself on a daily basis), I start off thinking about all the nutrient-dense veggies I'm going to add. This is not one of those recipes. I created this dish purely because I wanted something tasty. Still, these tacos contain a solid amount of fiber, protein, and omega-3 fatty acids. Not too shabby.

While I enjoy these tacos without sauce, they're also pretty tasty topped with either vegan ranch or "blue cheese" dressing. I know, "vegan blue cheese"—what a time to be alive.

YIELD: 6 small tacos (3 per serving)   PREP TIME: 5 minutes (not including time to make buttery spread or tortillas)   COOK TIME: 12 minutes

2 tablespoons (28g) Keto Buttery Spread (page 187) or vegan butter substitute of choice

¼ cup (60 ml) hot sauce

2 cups (280g) young green jackfruit, drained

1 recipe Flax Tortillas (page 180)

½ cup (50g) sliced celery

2 scallions (green parts only), sliced

- Heat the buttery spread and hot sauce in a small frying pan over medium heat until melted together. Add the jackfruit.

- Using a fork, mash the jackfruit to break up and separate the larger pieces; it should become almost stringy. You basically want it to look like shredded chicken.

- Stir to coat the jackfruit with the sauce. Continue to cook for about 10 minutes, until the jackfruit has absorbed all the sauce.

- To serve, divide the jackfruit mixture evenly among the 6 tortillas. Top with the celery and scallions.

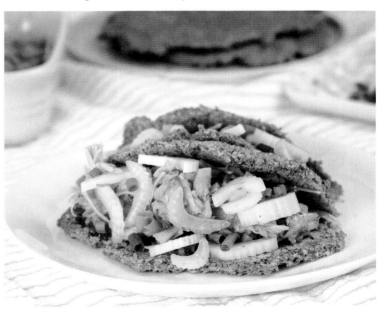

To store **Refrigerate the jackfruit mixture and tortillas in separate tightly sealed containers. The jackfruit mixture will keep for up to 3 days. The leftovers are best eaten cold.**

NUTRITION INFORMATION: **432** calories | **31.8g** fat | **11.2g** protein | **29.1g** total carbs | **5.4g** net carbs

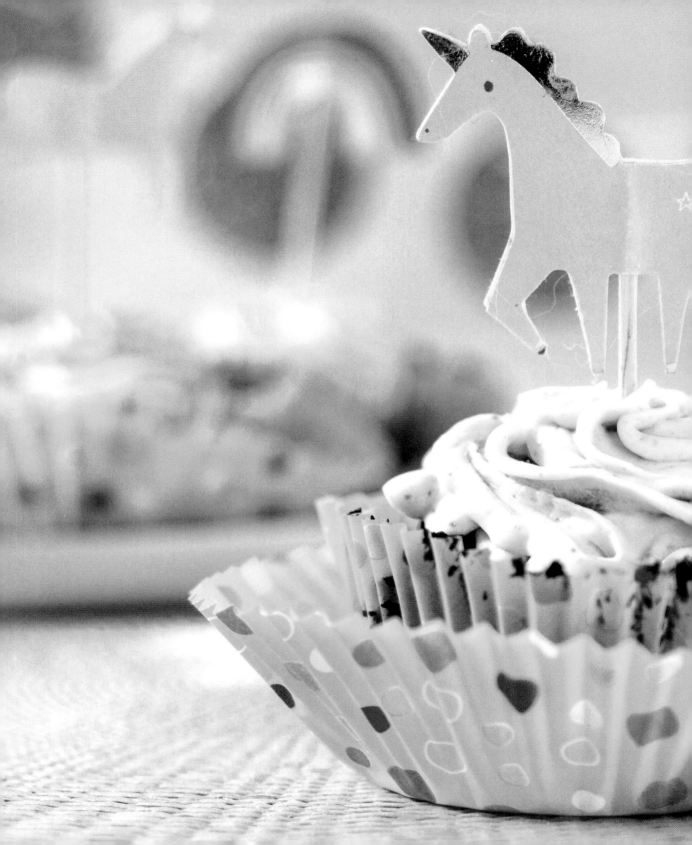

Drinks & Desserts

Sparkling Ginger Limeade

This light, refreshing beverage is a nonalcoholic take on my favorite happy hour indulgence—the Moscow Mule. It pairs nicely with a salad and is perfect for sipping on a hot summer day. If you're feeling fancy, garnish your drink with slices of lime and ginger and a sprig of mint.

   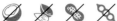

YIELD: four 10-ounce (300-ml) servings   PREP TIME: 10 minutes

¼ cup (60 ml) lime juice

2 teaspoons grated fresh ginger

1 (1-L) bottle plain seltzer water

3 or 4 drops liquid stevia (optional)

Ice cubes, for serving

FOR GARNISH (OPTIONAL):

4 lime slices

4 ginger slices

4 fresh mint sprigs

- In a 1-quart (1-L) pitcher or jar, stir together the lime juice and ginger.

- Pour in the seltzer water. Add the stevia, if using, and stir to combine.

- Fill four 10-ounce (300-ml) glasses with ice.

- Divide the limeade among the glasses. If desired, garnish each serving with a lime slice, ginger slice, and sprig of mint.

Note: **Because of the seltzer, this drink is best served fresh.**

NUTRITION INFORMATION: **5** calories | **0g** fat | **0g** protein | **1.7g** total carbs | **1.6g** net carbs

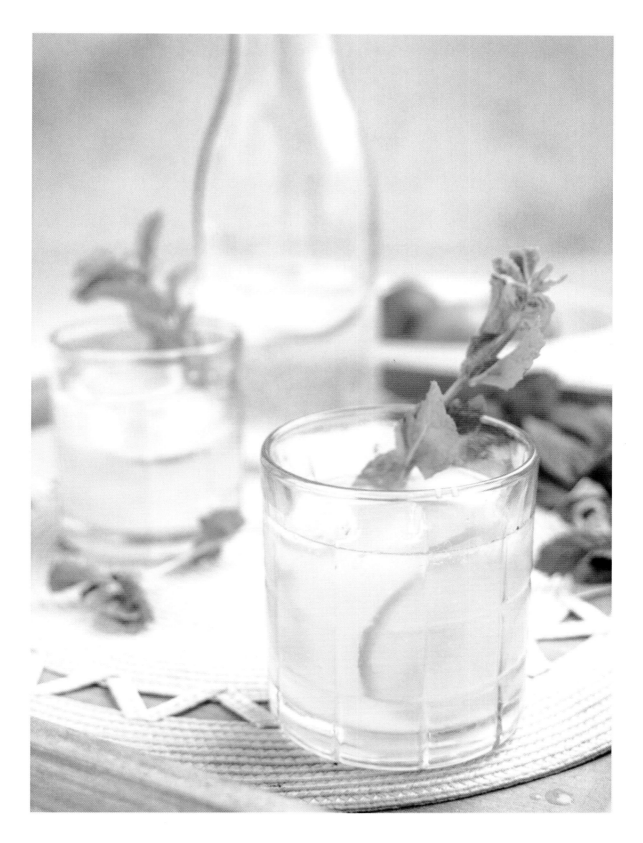

Blackberry Lemonade

I pretty routinely make myself a lazy "keto lemonade" with just lemon juice, water, and sometimes stevia. But when I want to treat myself, I whip up a batch of this blackberry lemonade. Lightly sweet and tangy, it is a great way to sneak in some extra antioxidants. This recipe works really well with raspberries, too!

  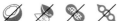

YIELD: four 10-ounce (300-ml) servings   PREP TIME: 10 minutes

½ cup (70g) blackberries

¼ cup (60 ml) lemon juice

4 cups (1L) water, divided

4 or 5 drops liquid stevia (optional)

Ice, for serving

FOR GARNISH (OPTIONAL):

8 lemon slices

8 blackberries

4 fresh mint sprigs

- Put the blackberries and lemon juice in a blender with 1 cup (240 ml) of the water and blend just long enough to extract the juice from the blackberries, about 10 seconds.

- Strain the mixture into a pitcher, then add the remaining 3 cups (710 ml) of water and the stevia, if using, and stir.

- Fill four 10-ounce (300-ml) glasses with ice.

- Divide the lemonade among the glasses. If desired, garnish each glass with a couple of lemon slices, a couple of blackberries, and a sprig of mint.

To store **Refrigerate in a tightly sealed container, separate from garnishes, for up to 3 days.**

NUTRITION INFORMATION: **6** calories | **0.1g** fat | **0.1g** protein | **1.7g** total carbs | **1.6g** net carbs

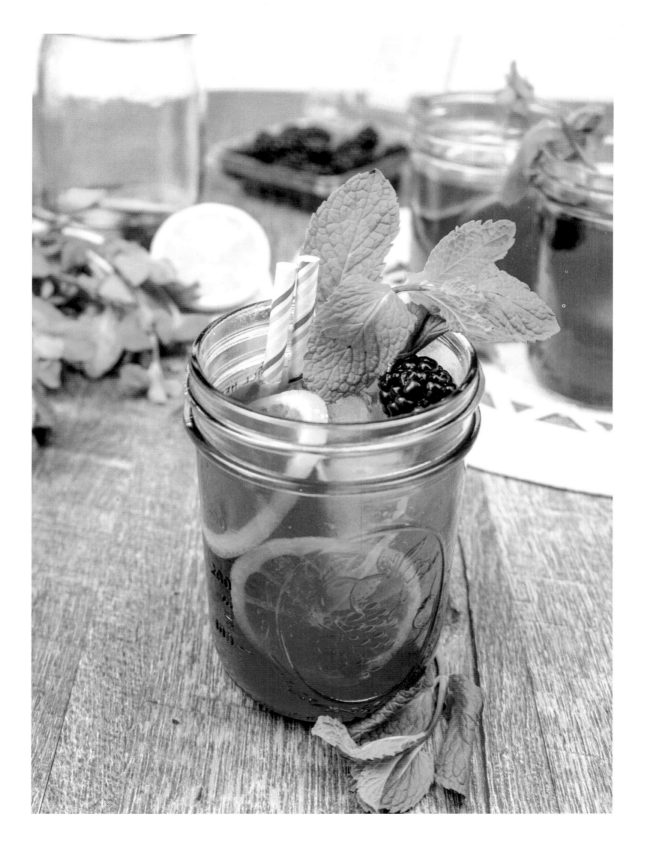

Coconut Matcha Latte

The first time I tried matcha, I was working as a barista while studying nutrition, and I was immediately hooked. At the time, fatty coffees were becoming more mainstream, so it only seemed natural to adapt matcha lattes to be keto-friendly, too.

There are two main grades of matcha: ceremonial and culinary. The ceremonial grade is pretty spendy, so I stick with the culinary, especially since I always combine matcha with other ingredients that would mask the more refined flavor of ceremonial-grade matcha.

YIELD: four 8-ounce (240-ml) servings
PREP TIME: 5 minutes   COOK TIME: 5 minutes

1½ cups (360 ml) pea milk or other nondairy milk of choice, divided

2 rounded teaspoons matcha green tea powder, plus extra for sprinkling

1 (13.5-ounce/400-ml) can full-fat coconut milk

1½ teaspoons vanilla extract

10 drops liquid stevia

- In a small mixing bowl, whisk together ¼ cup (60 ml) of the pea milk with the matcha powder until smooth and free of lumps.

- Pour the milk mixture into a small saucepan along with the remaining 1¼ cups (300 ml) of pea milk and the coconut milk. Stir to combine. Bring to a simmer over medium heat.

- Remove the pan from the heat, stir in the vanilla extract and stevia, and pour into teacups. Sprinkle with a little matcha and serve.

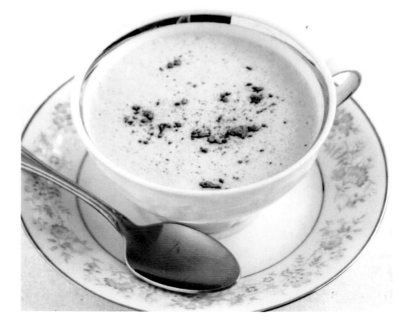

To store Refrigerate in a tightly sealed jar for up to 5 days.

To reheat Bring the tea mixture to a simmer in a saucepan over medium heat, stirring frequently.

Note Replace the vanilla extract with peppermint extract or raspberry extract for a totally different flavor.

NUTRITION INFORMATION: **183** calories | **15.5g** fat | **4.9g** protein | **3.3g** total carbs | **3.3g** net carbs

Keto Pumpkin Spice Latte

Every fall, I'm bombarded with advertisements for pumpkin spice lattes, and every fall, a part of me is actually tempted to indulge in one of those sugar bombs. Instead, I came up with this homemade version to satisfy that craving in a more nutrient-dense way. Is this a traditional latte? No, but it sure does satisfy that craving (while packing a solid amount of protein)!

YIELD: 1 serving (about 12 ounces/350 ml)
PREP TIME: 3 minutes   COOK TIME: 5 minutes

1 cup (240 ml) brewed coffee

¹/₃ cup (80 ml) canned full-fat coconut milk

2 tablespoons (30g) pumpkin puree

2 tablespoons (14g) pea protein powder or other vegan protein powder of choice

1 teaspoon Chai Spice Blend (page 173) or ground cinnamon

10 drops liquid stevia

Ground cinnamon, for sprinkling

- Place all the ingredients in a small saucepan over low heat. Heat for about 5 minutes, whisking occasionally, until the desired temperature is reached.

- Carefully pour the latte into a mug and sprinkle with a little cinnamon to enjoy.

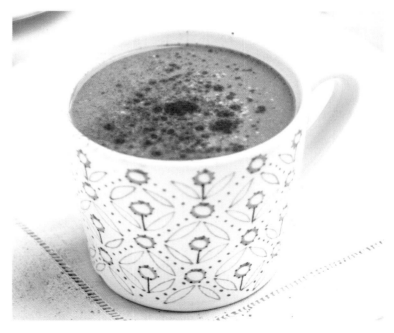

Tip *Freeze the remaining pumpkin puree in an ice cube tray in 2-tablespoon portions, then use them as needed for future lattes. This works especially well for making Iced Pumpkin Spice Lattes.*

Variation ICED PUMPKIN SPICE LATTE. *Fill a pint glass or jar (475 ml) with ice. Use a blender to blend the latte ingredients, then pour over the ice to serve.*

NUTRITION INFORMATION: **199** calories | **13.6g** fat | **12.6g** protein | **5.6g** total carbs | **3.5g** net carbs

Golden Chai Protein Smoothie

This anti-inflammatory protein smoothie is a perfect pre- or post-workout treat.

Curcumin, the most studied anti-inflammatory compound in turmeric, is best absorbed when consumed with piperine, a compound found in black pepper. If you use a store-bought chai spice blend that doesn't contain black pepper, try adding a few grinds to the blender with the other spices.

   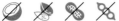

YIELD: two 10-ounce (300-ml) servings   PREP TIME: 3 minutes

2 cups (480 ml) pea milk or other nondairy milk of choice

1 medium Hass avocado (7½ ounces/212g), peeled and pitted

¼ cup (28g) pea protein powder or other vegan protein powder of choice

1½ teaspoons Chai Spice Blend (page 173), plus extra for sprinkling

1 teaspoon turmeric powder

⅛ teaspoon liquid stevia

- Put all the ingredients in a blender and blend until completely smooth, 30 to 60 seconds.

- Pour the smoothie into 2 glasses or jars, sprinkle a little more chai spice on top, and enjoy!

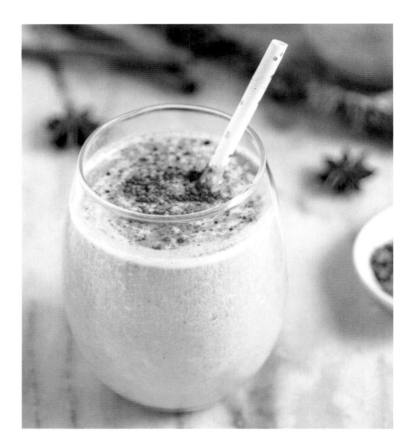

To store Refrigerate in a tightly sealed jar for up to 2 days.

NUTRITION INFORMATION: **250** calories | **15.9g** fat | **21.6g** protein | **9.5g** total carbs | **3.1g** net carbs

Rise & Shine Smoothie

In late spring and summer, when it's really warm out, I tend to enjoy smoothies a bit more often. They're a great way to sneak in some protein and greens without having to touch the stovetop. This is my favorite smoothie. It has so much protein from whole-food sources, as well as omega-3 fatty acids. Plus, it's just so tasty!

I'm a little weird in that I don't really like cold things, so I don't add ice to this smoothie, but you could add some ice cubes to the blender to make it colder if you prefer.

 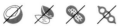

YIELD: one 16-ounce (475-ml) serving   PREP TIME: 5 minutes

1 cup (240 ml) water or nondairy milk of choice

2 lightly packed cups (60g) fresh spinach

¼ cup (40g) hulled hemp seeds

2 tablespoons (14g) ground flax seeds

1 packed tablespoon fresh mint leaves

1 tablespoon lemon juice

¼ teaspoon vanilla extract

Ice (optional)

Fresh mint sprig, for garnish (optional)

Put all the ingredients in a blender and blend until completely smooth, 2 to 3 minutes. Pour into a pint glass or jar (475 ml) to serve. Garnish with a fresh mint sprig, if desired.

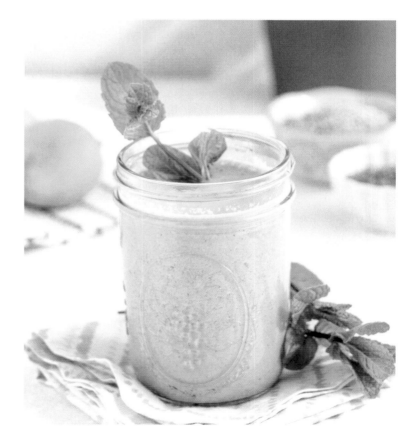

Note If you don't love lemon flavor, you can substitute lime juice or even ½ teaspoon of raspberry or mint extract.

Tip A friend of mine swears by this trick for making chilled green smoothies: Blend up a bunch of spinach and pour it into ice cube trays. Once frozen, transfer the cubes to a zip-top freezer bag and use as needed for smoothies.

NUTRITION INFORMATION: **322** calories | **23.5g** fat | **17.7g** protein | **11.5g** total carbs | **2.2g** net carbs

Chocolate Almond Butter Cupcakes

This is one of those recipes that came about by accident. In an attempt to make chocolate pancakes, it became apparent that the batter would be put to much better use for cupcakes. I was tempted to call these "brownie cakes" because they have a wonderfully dense texture, sort of like a cakey brownie. I make these at least once a week—they are so easy to throw together and are absolutely perfect with a glass of coconut milk.

You can make these cupcakes nut-free by replacing the almond butter with tahini or sunflower seed butter and the almond milk with coconut milk.

YIELD: 4 cupcakes (1 per serving)
PREP TIME: 15 minutes, plus time to cool   COOK TIME: 30 minutes

CUPCAKES:

¼ cup (64g) unsweetened creamy almond butter, room temperature

¼ cup (60 ml) unsweetened almond milk or other nondairy milk of choice

2 tablespoons (24g) granulated sweetener

2 tablespoons (14g) ground flax seeds

2 rounded tablespoons (20g) cocoa powder

½ teaspoon baking powder

FROSTING:

⅓ cup (80g) coconut cream (see Note)

1 tablespoon unsweetened creamy almond butter, room temperature

- Preheat the oven to 350°F (177°C). Line 4 wells of a standard-size muffin pan with paper liners or have a standard-size silicone muffin pan on hand.

- In a small mixing bowl, whisk together the almond butter and almond milk until well combined and smooth. Stir in the sweetener and flax seeds and set aside.

- In a separate bowl, whisk together the cocoa powder and baking powder until thoroughly combined.

- Fold the dry ingredients into the wet, then continue to stir until no lumps remain.

- Divide the batter evenly among the 4 lined muffin wells (or 4 wells of the silicone pan), filling each about three-quarters full. Bake for 30 minutes, or until firm to the touch.

- Remove from the oven and let cool in the pan for at least 20 minutes to allow the cupcakes to set up. Remove from the pan and allow to cool completely before frosting.

- To make the frosting, place the coconut cream in a small mixing bowl. Stir in the almond butter.

- Once the cupcakes have cooled completely, frost and enjoy.

To store **These cupcakes will keep covered at room temperature for up to 2 days (3 days if unfrosted), or up to 5 days if kept in a tightly sealed container in the fridge.**

Note *To get coconut cream, chill a can of full-fat coconut milk in the refrigerator for at least 4 hours. Open the can and scoop out the thick, solid "cream" that has risen to the top two-thirds of the can. One can should yield about 1 cup (240g) of cream. Discard the liquid at the bottom of the can or use it in smoothies. The cream will keep in a tightly sealed container in the refrigerator for up to 3 days.*

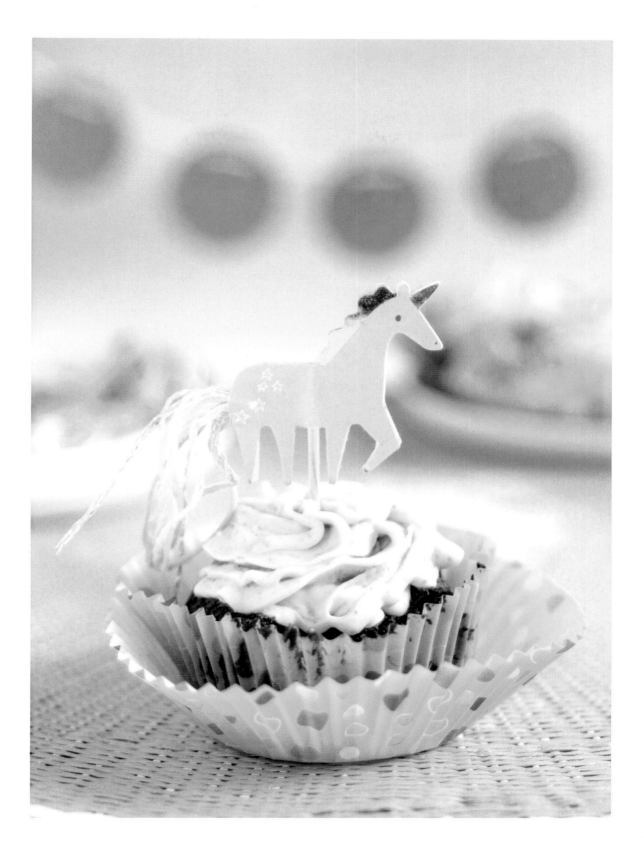

Keto Black Bean Brownies

Remember the joy you experienced when you first tasted a black bean brownie? They're brownies made of beans, and they're actually delicious. They're pretty darn close to perfection with one minor caveat—all the sugar and carbs. These black bean brownies are made with black soybeans and eschew sugar in favor of a granulated sweetener that won't spike your blood glucose. It's having your cake and eating it, too.

YIELD: 9 brownies (1 per serving)   PREP TIME: 5 minutes
COOK TIME: 40 minutes

1 (15-ounce/425-g) can unsalted black soybeans, drained and rinsed

½ cup (132g) tahini, room temperature

¼ heaping cup (40g) cocoa powder

¼ cup (48g) granulated sweetener

1 teaspoon vanilla extract

½ teaspoon baking powder

¼ teaspoon salt

- Preheat the oven to 350°F (177°C) and line an 8-inch (20-cm) square baking pan with parchment. Leave at least 2 inches (5 cm) of extra parchment on two opposite sides to help with removal later.

- Put all the ingredients in a blender or food processor and blend until smooth, about 90 seconds.

- The batter will be too thick to pour but will spread easily. Scoop the batter into the lined pan and spread it out in an even layer.

- Bake for 40 minutes, until the top is firm to the touch and a toothpick inserted in the center comes out clean.

- Remove from the oven and let cool in the pan for about 5 minutes before removing. To remove, grasp the overhanging parchment and gently lift the brownies out of the pan. Let cool completely before slicing and serving.

To store **Store in a sealed container at room temperature for up to 3 days or in the refrigerator for up to 5 days.**

To reheat **While these brownies are delicious cold, placing them in a preheated 300°F (150°C) oven for 5 minutes will warm them nicely.**

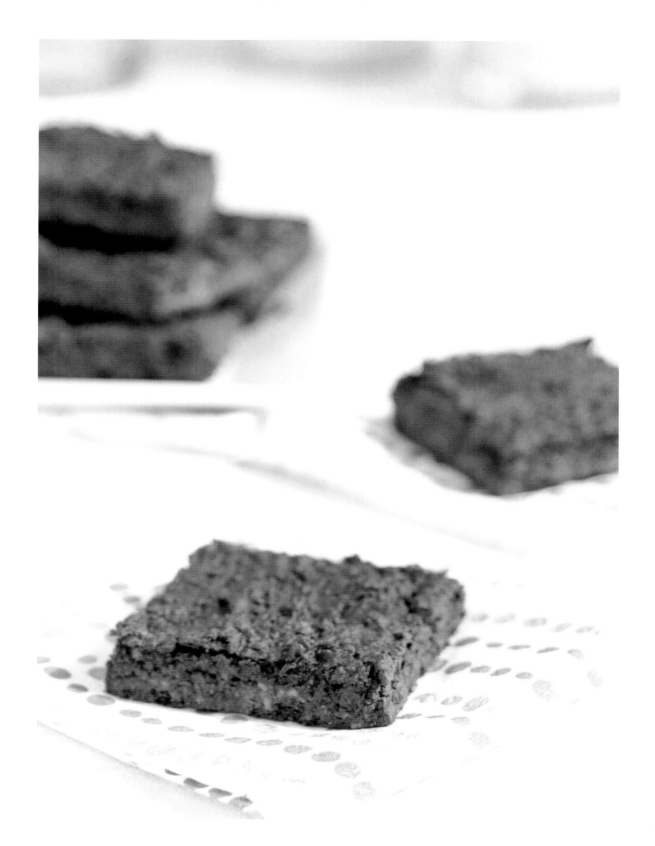

Chocolate Keto Nice Cream

When I ate a high-carb vegan diet, nice cream made with bananas was a staple. After starting keto, I figured nice cream was one of those treats I would have to leave behind. There are some tasty low-carb vegan ice cream options sold in stores now, but they're not super widely available.

This recipe makes a rich, smooth nice cream that doesn't require an ice cream maker. It also provides a lot of healthy fats and other micronutrients. So it's basically a health food . . .

YIELD: about 1 pint (440g) (4 servings)
PREP TIME: 5 minutes, plus time to freeze

1 cup (240g) coconut cream (see Note, page 162)

1 medium Hass avocado (7½ ounces/212g), peeled and pitted

¼ heaping cup (40g) cocoa powder

¼ cup (48g) powdered sweetener

1 teaspoon vanilla extract

SUGGESTED TOPPINGS:

Toasted unsweetened coconut flakes

Cacao nibs

- Put all the ingredients in a blender or food processor and blend until smooth, about 90 seconds.

- Pour the mixture into an airtight container and freeze for 4 to 6 hours, until firm and scoopable.

- Serve and enjoy, topped with coconut flakes and/or cacao nibs, if desired.

To store Freeze in a tightly sealed container for up to 2 weeks.

To soften This nice cream freezes pretty hard. If it's been in the freezer for more than 6 hours, you might need to leave it on the counter to soften for about a half hour before serving.

Tip If you have a super-powerful blender, cube and freeze the avocado before blending everything. This will make a soft serve–like nice cream that can be enjoyed immediately!

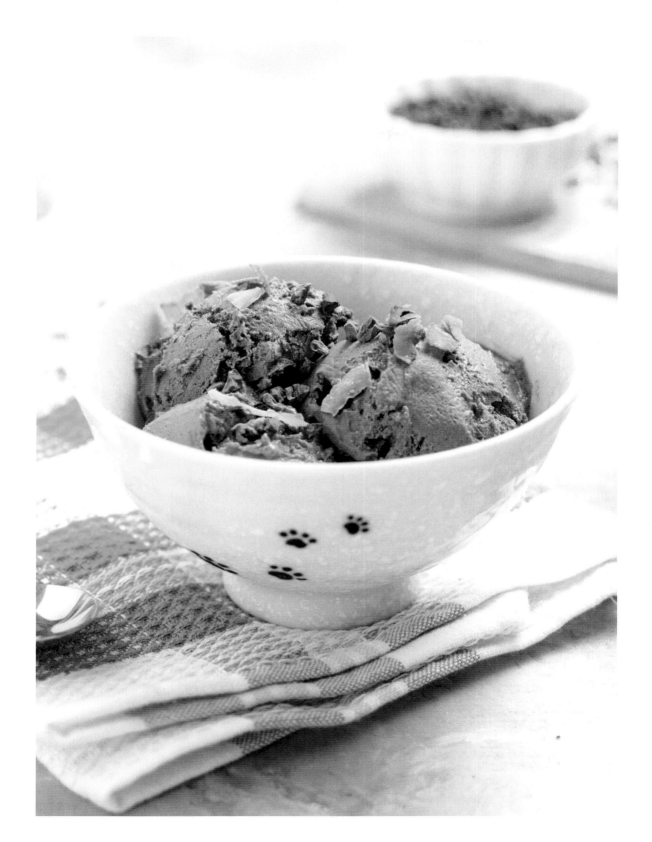

Snickerdoodles

If I had to choose a favorite cookie, the winner (by far) would be snickerdoodles. So rich and full of delicious cinnamon flavor, how could a person not love them? These cookies come together quickly and satisfy that need for a cinnamon-y treat. They're slightly chewy and taste delicious with a cup of coffee.

¼ cup (28g) ground flax seeds

1 teaspoon ground cinnamon, plus extra for dusting if desired

½ teaspoon baking powder

½ cup (128g) unsweetened creamy almond butter, room temperature

2 Flax Eggs (page 182)

2 tablespoons (30 ml) unsweetened coconut milk or other nondairy milk of choice

¼ cup (48g) granulated sweetener

1 teaspoon vanilla extract

YIELD: 10 cookies (1 per serving)
PREP TIME: 10 minutes   COOK TIME: 25 minutes

- Preheat the oven to 350°F (177°C) and line a cookie sheet with parchment paper.

- In a small bowl, whisk together the flax seeds, cinnamon, and baking powder.

- In a medium-sized bowl, stir together the almond butter, flax eggs, nondairy milk, sweetener, and vanilla extract.

- Stir the dry ingredients into the wet until a smooth dough forms. It should have the consistency of a drop-cookie dough.

- Using a spoon, scoop the dough onto the lined cookie sheet to make 10 cookies, about 2 tablespoons (30 ml) each. Space the cookies about 1 inch (2.5 cm) apart. Smooth out any jagged edges so they don't overcook before spreading. If desired, dust the tops with cinnamon.

- Bake for 25 minutes, until the tops are firm to the touch.

- Remove from the oven and transfer to a cooling rack with a spatula. Allow to cool and set up for at least 15 minutes before eating.

To store Store in a covered container at room temperature for up to 4 days.

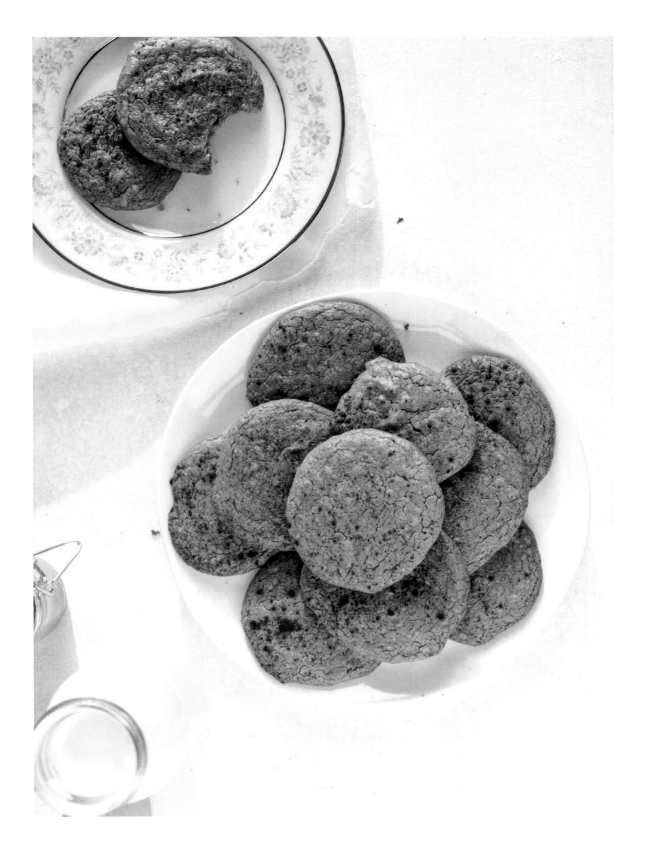

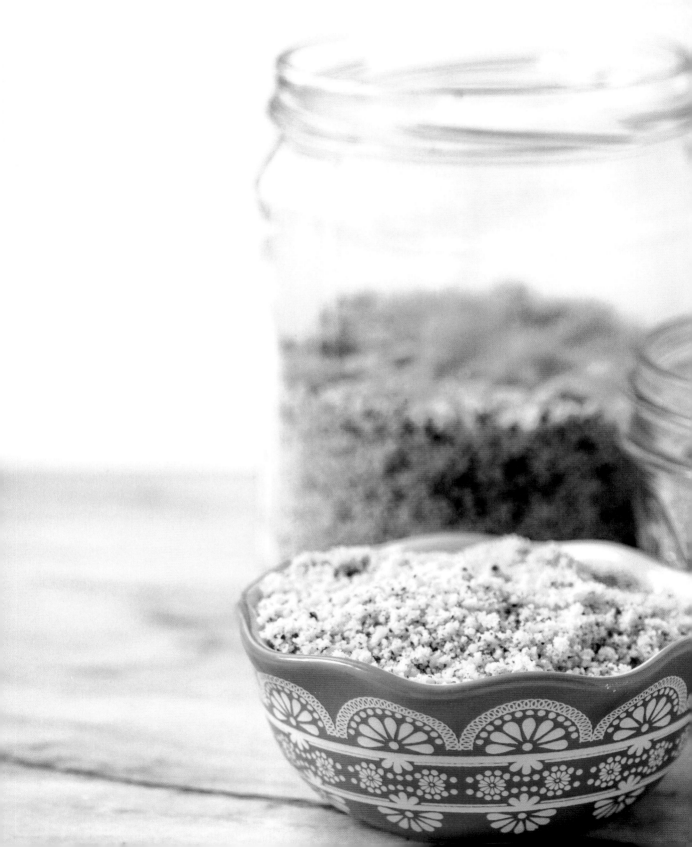

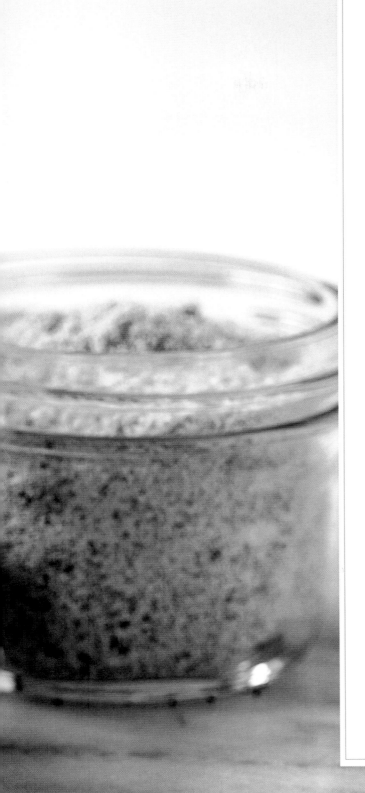

Basics

Sausage Spice Blend

I couldn't tell you why, but I found myself craving sausage one day—not necessarily the sausage itself, but the herbs and spices that combine to make sausage. This blend is a hybrid of various recipes I've come across over the years, and it has that flavor combination I'm looking for. I use it to make my Sausage-Style Breakfast Patties (page 64).

  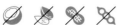

YIELD: about ¼ cup (25g)   PREP TIME: 5 minutes

2 tablespoons dried parsley leaves

2 teaspoons dried thyme leaves

2 teaspoons fennel seeds

2 teaspoons granulated garlic

1 teaspoon ground black pepper

½ teaspoon paprika

½ teaspoon red pepper flakes

Put the ingredients in a tightly lidded container and shake to combine. Store tightly sealed, away from heat and light, for up to 3 months.

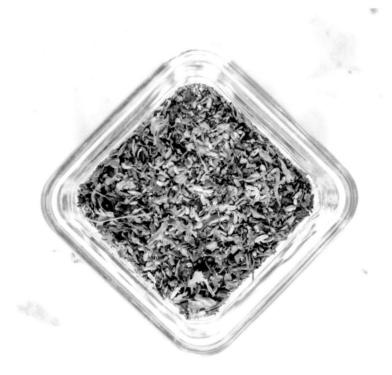

Variation BREAKFAST SAUSAGE BLEND. *To the ingredients above, add 1 tablespoon of dried rubbed sage and 1 tablespoon of granulated sweetener.*

Chai Spice Blend

There's something so pleasant and warming about anything flavored with chai spices. The word *chai* actually just means "tea," but it has become synonymous with the seasoning blends containing varying amounts of the spices below. There are tons of different chai spice blends out there, and this one is the one that I have come to use over the years. You can tweak it however you like to suit your tastes!

The best cup of chai tea I ever had was made by my cousin-in-law's mother, who was from Punjab. I haven't yet had another cup that was so rich and delicious, but anytime I use this spice blend, I'm reminded of that day.

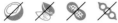

YIELD: ¼ cup (30g)   PREP TIME: 5 minutes

1 tablespoon plus 1 teaspoon ground cinnamon

1 tablespoon ground cardamom

2 teaspoons ginger powder

1 teaspoon ground anise seed

1 teaspoon ground cloves

1 teaspoon ground nutmeg

½ teaspoon ground black pepper

Put the ingredients in a tightly lidded container and shake to combine. Store tightly sealed, away from heat and light, for up to 3 months.

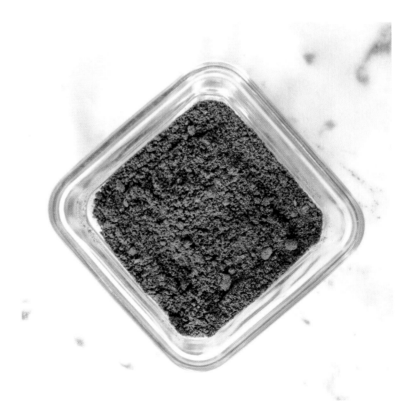

Everything Bagel Blend

This blend was inspired by a store-bought blend with a similar name. I was running low one day and realized that I could just make my own, refill the shaker, and save myself a trip to the store. My husband didn't even notice the difference, which I think is a big win.

   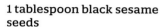

YIELD: about ¼ cup (30g)   PREP TIME: 5 minutes

1 tablespoon black sesame seeds

1 tablespoon white sesame seeds

1 tablespoon dehydrated onion flakes

1½ teaspoons granulated garlic

1½ teaspoons kosher salt

Put the ingredients in a tightly lidded container and shake to combine. Store tightly sealed, away from heat and light, for up to 3 months.

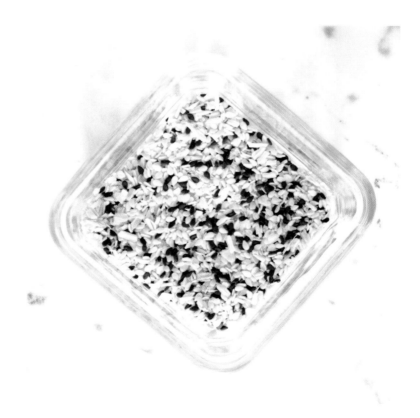

Savory Herb Blend

I use this herb blend in just about everything, from soups and pot pies to breakfast scrambles.

   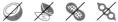

YIELD: ½ cup (25g)   PREP TIME: 5 minutes

2 tablespoons dehydrated onion flakes

2 tablespoons dried thyme leaves

1 tablespoon plus 1 teaspoon dried marjoram leaves

1 tablespoon plus 1 teaspoon dried rubbed sage

1 tablespoon plus 1 teaspoon granulated garlic

Put the ingredients in a tightly lidded container and shake to combine. Store tightly sealed, away from heat and light, for up to 3 months.

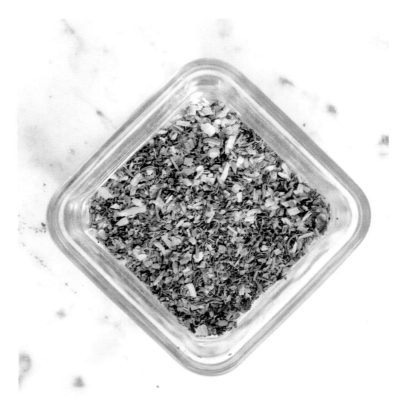

Nut & Seed Flours

I like to make my own nut and seed flours both to save money and to have access to fresher flours. After a nut or seed is ground, it starts oxidizing (going rancid) much faster than if it were left whole. Making nut flours on an as-needed basis, or at least in smaller batches, helps ensure that your flours won't spoil before you can use them. Grinding your own flours also gives you more flexibility. For instance, if you can't tolerate nuts, you often can substitute an equal amount of sunflower seed flour for the almond flour in a recipe.

Nuts and seeds that work really well for making flours include almonds, hazelnuts, pecans, walnuts, sunflower seeds, and hemp seeds. These are all low in carbs and add interesting flavors wherever you use them.

 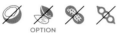
OPTION

Hulled raw nuts or seeds of choice (see Notes)

YIELD: varies   PREP TIME: 5 minutes

- Put the nuts or seeds in a food processor or high-powered blender and process until they are ground into a flour. If the flour starts to look oily or clump at all, stop the blender or food processor immediately, or you will end up with nut or seed butter.

- Sift out the larger pieces of nuts or seeds and process again until the flour is uniform.

To use Replace the almond flour called for in a recipe with an equal amount of homemade nut or seed flour. To replace coconut flour, use 3 times as much nut or seed flour, adding more if the dough/batter still looks too wet.

To store Store in a tightly lidded container away from heat and light for up to a week, refrigerate for up to 2 weeks, or freeze for up to a month.

Notes The quantity of nuts or seeds to use here really depends on the recipe you are making with the nut or seed flour. I usually weigh out the amount of nuts or seeds I need based on the weight of the flour called for in the recipe and then grind that amount.

For a more refined flour, I often buy blanched almonds or hazelnuts that already have the outer skins removed. This gives the flour more of a traditional appearance, as it will be uniform in color.

Some blenders or food processors work best when there is a certain volume of ingredients in the container, so keep this in mind when making flour. You may need to grind a bit more than your recipe calls for.

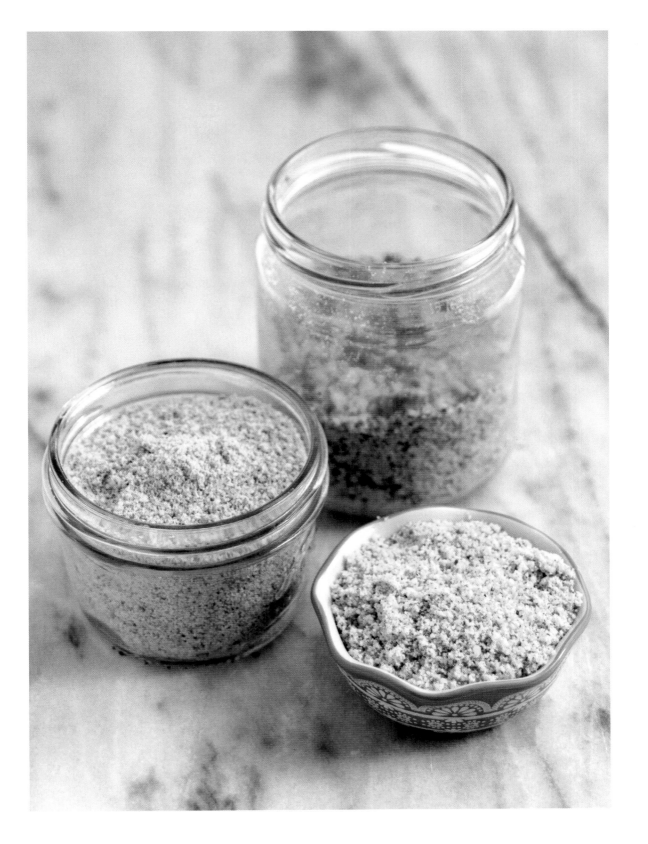

Cauliflower Rice

Thanks to the popularity of the Paleo diet, you can buy fresh or frozen cauliflower rice pretty much anywhere. However, I tend to make my own when cauliflower is in season, as it is more cost-effective and fresher-tasting. I find it easier to chop the cauliflower florets and stalk into smaller pieces before processing; otherwise, the resulting "grains" aren't uniform in size and won't cook evenly.

5½ cups (565g) coarsely chopped cauliflower (florets and stem from 1 medium head of cauliflower, about 5 inches/ 13 cm in diameter)

YIELD: about 5 cups (565g)   PREP TIME: 5 minutes

- Process the cauliflower pieces in a blender or food processor until they are about twice the size of grains of rice. If the pieces are too small, they can be difficult to work with in recipes and may become mushy.

- Use in recipes as directed, or follow the instructions below to cook.

To store **Refrigerate raw cauliflower rice in a tightly sealed container for up to 5 days or freeze for up to a month.**

To cook **I like to steam my cauliflower rice with 2 to 3 tablespoons of water and a pinch of salt in a large covered frying pan over medium heat for about 10 minutes, stirring occasionally, until the rice softens. If the water evaporates too quickly, add another 1 to 2 tablespoons.**

Variation PESTO CAULIFLOWER RICE. **In a medium-sized frying pan, stir together 4 cups (452g) of uncooked cauliflower rice and ⅔ cup (160 ml) of Easy Vegan Pesto (page 189). Cover with the lid and cook over medium heat for 10 minutes, stirring occasionally, until the rice softens.**

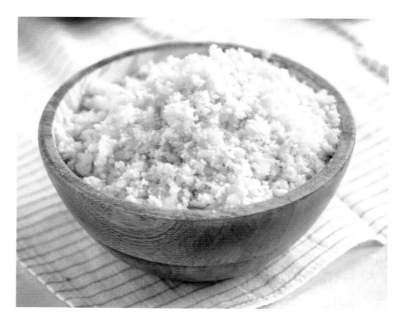

NUTRITION INFORMATION (per cup/113g): **28** calories | **0.3g** fat | **2.1g** protein | **5.7g** total carbs | **3.4g** net carbs

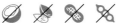

Zucchini Noodles

I put off buying a spiral slicer for a long time, thinking I didn't want yet another gadget cluttering my kitchen. I'm so glad I finally took the plunge. I had been making noodles with my mandoline slicer, and the spiral slicer is much faster. I just have a small handheld spiral slicer, but you also can buy a larger model that sits on your countertop.

If you become bored with zucchini noodles, you can try spiral-slicing other vegetables. I like using spiral-sliced cucumber in salads instead of round slices. I've also had success spiralizing carrots, parsnips, and daikon radishes—pretty much any long, cylindrical vegetable will work.

3 small zucchini (3½ ounces/ 100g each)

YIELD: about 2 cups (200g)   PREP TIME: 5 minutes

- If using a spiral slicer, make the zucchini noodles according to the directions that came with your slicer.

- If you are using a mandoline slicer, set it to the julienne setting and place it securely over the rim of a medium-sized mixing bowl. (If your mandoline came with an attachable tray to catch the slices, use that instead.) Secure the hand guard that came with the slicer onto the zucchini and drag the zucchini lengthwise over the blade to create noodles.

- Cook according to the recipe directions, or follow the instructions below.

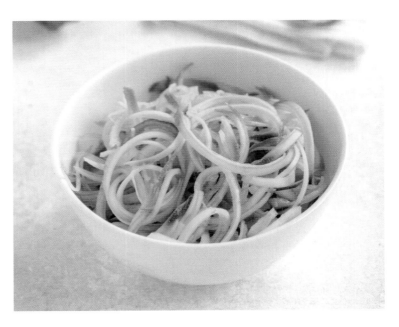

To store Refrigerate raw zucchini noodles in a tightly sealed container for up to 3 days.

To cook Place the zucchini noodles and 1 to 2 tablespoons of water or olive oil in a medium-sized frying pan over medium heat. Cover with the lid and cook for 3 to 5 minutes, until the noodles reach the desired tenderness.

Tip You can use pretty much any summer squash variety in place of the zucchini.

NUTRITION INFORMATION (per cup/100g): **17** calories | **0.3g** fat | **1.2g** protein | **3.1g** total carbs | **2.1g** net carbs

Flax Tortillas

Perfecting the technique of making these flax tortillas takes a little bit of practice, but once you get the hang of it, you'll be making them all the time! When made into 4-inch (10-cm) tortillas, they work great as taco shells, but you can make them larger for use as wraps (see the Variation below).

  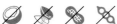

YIELD: six 4-inch (10-cm) tortillas (2 per serving)
PREP TIME: 10 minutes   COOK TIME: 18 minutes

1 cup (112g) ground flax seeds

½ cup (120 ml) water

¼ teaspoon salt

- Place a medium-sized nonstick frying pan over medium-low heat.

- In a bowl, mix together the flax seeds, water, and salt. Let sit for a few minutes until a thick, slightly sticky dough forms. Divide the dough into 6 equal portions, then shape each portion into a ball.

- To cook each tortilla, place a dough ball in the hot frying pan and use a fork or spatula to gently flatten it into a 4-inch (10-cm) round. Cook until the tortilla is set on top and you can shimmy a spatula under it without disturbing the shape, about 2 minutes. Flip and cook for 1 minute on the other side. Repeat with the remaining dough balls.

To store Tightly wrap and refrigerate for up to a week or freeze for up to a month.

To reheat While leftovers can be enjoyed cold (I prefer them that way!), the tortillas can be warmed in a preheated 300°F (150°C) oven for 5 minutes or until the desired temperature is reached.

Variation FLAX WRAPS. *To make 6-inch (15-cm) flax tortillas that are great for wraps, use a 10-inch (25-cm) or larger frying pan and divide the dough into three equal portions instead of six. Place a dough ball in the preheated frying pan and flatten it as described above into a 5-inch (13-cm) round. Cook it on both sides as described above, then remove the wrap from the pan and immediately roll it out on a clean work surface to 6 inches (15 cm).*

NUTRITION INFORMATION: **199** calories | **15.7g** fat | **6.8g** protein | **10.8g** total carbs | **0.6g** net carbs

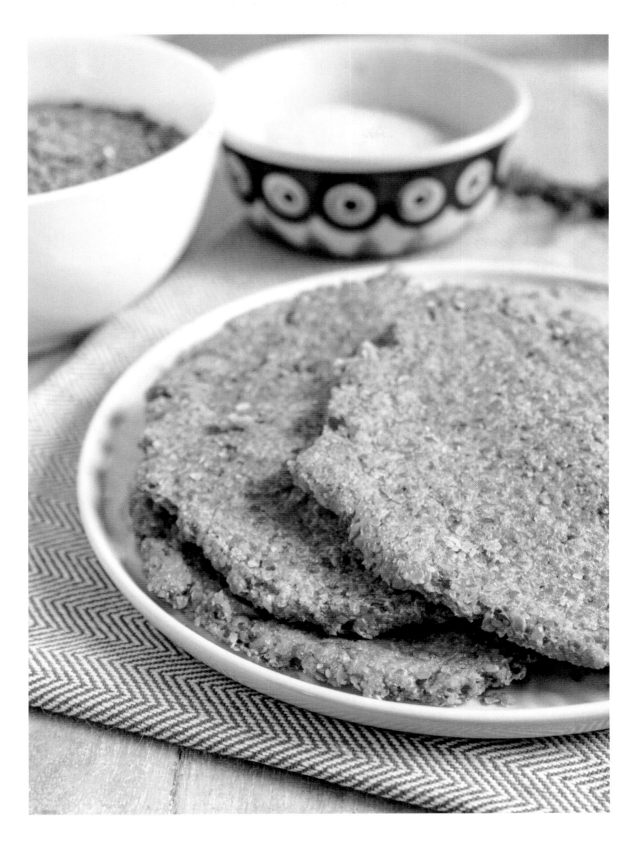

Flax Egg

Flax eggs are a great binder in recipes where an egg would normally hold ingredients together, like cookies or the filling in a cabbage roll. If you are unable to tolerate flax, an equal measure of ground chia seeds also works. The reason for making the flax egg 5 minutes ahead of time is to allow a gel to form, which is what creates that binding power.

While flax eggs are pretty versatile, there are some instances where they really don't work as an egg substitute—basically anywhere the egg is used for volume, like in a soufflé, quiche, or angel food cake.

  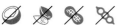

YIELD: 1 flax egg   PREP TIME: 5 minutes

3 tablespoons (45 ml) water

1 tablespoon ground flax seeds

- Whisk together the water and flax seeds in a small dish. Set aside for 5 minutes, until the mixture has thickened somewhat and lightened in color.

- Use immediately in place of one egg as directed in the recipe you are making.

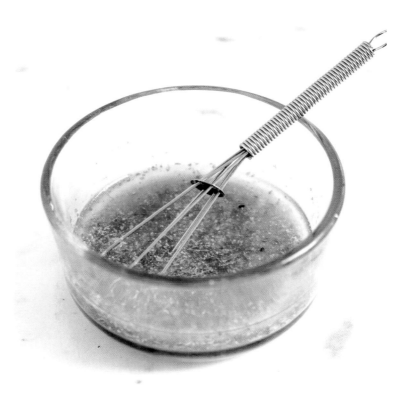

NUTRITION INFORMATION: **37** calories | **3g** fat | **1.3g** protein | **2g** total carbs | **0.1g** net carbs

Tangy Avocado Mayo

Who would have thought that mayo was so easy to make? This delicious and creamy version uses the all-star fruit and keto darling, the avocado, as a base, so you can sneak some B vitamins and potassium into everything you eat.

   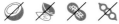

YIELD: about 1 cup (240 ml) (1 tablespoon per serving)
PREP TIME: 5 minutes

1 medium Hass avocado (7½ ounces/212g), peeled and pitted

¼ cup (60 ml) extra-virgin olive oil

Juice of 1 lime, or juice of ½ lemon

1 teaspoon Sriracha sauce or chili paste

Pinch of salt

Using a blender or food processor, blend all the ingredients until smooth and creamy, 15 to 30 seconds.

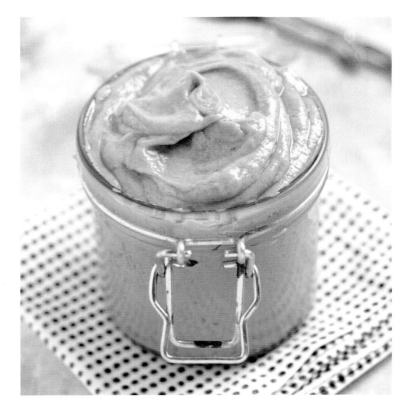

To store **Refrigerate in a tightly sealed jar for up to a week.**

Tip **If you overblend the mayo, it will start to look curdled. Blending in ½ to 1 teaspoon of pea protein powder will make it smooth and creamy again.**

NUTRITION INFORMATION: **45** calories | **4.7g** fat | **0.2g** protein | **1g** total carbs | **0.4g** net carbs

Easy Mustard Vinaigrette

Mustard is hands-down my favorite condiment, so it's only natural that I would want to turn it into a salad dressing. I like to make this dressing with either a spicy brown mustard or a German-style mustard for a little extra kick.

  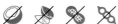

½ cup (120 ml) extra-virgin olive oil

¼ cup plus 2 tablespoons (90 ml) prepared mustard of choice

2 tablespoons (30 ml) apple cider vinegar

1 teaspoon crushed garlic

¼ teaspoon ground black pepper

YIELD: 1 cup (240 ml) (2 tablespoons/30 ml per serving)
PREP TIME: 3 minutes

Put all the ingredients in a tightly sealed jar and shake to emulsify.

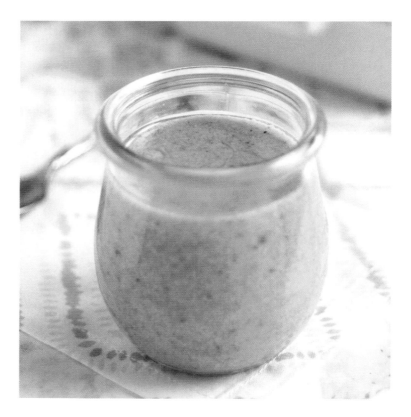

To store Refrigerate for up to 2 weeks.

Quick Hemp Seed Sour Cream

This sour "cream" whips up quickly and is a great soy-free alternative to the vegan sour cream products that are available in stores, which aren't very nutrient dense and often contain trans fats. It makes a great topping for my Meal Prep Chili (page 142).

   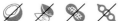 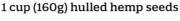

YIELD: about 1¼ cups (300 ml) (2 tablespoons/30 ml per serving)
PREP TIME: 3 minutes

1 cup (160g) hulled hemp seeds

¼ cup (60 ml) extra-virgin olive oil

¼ cup (60 ml) water

Juice of 1 lemon

¼ teaspoon salt

In a food processor or blender, blend all the ingredients until completely smooth, 1 to 2 minutes.

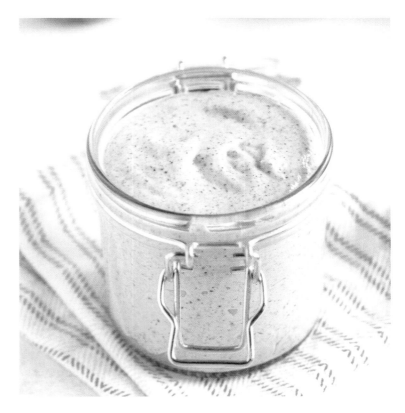

To store **Refrigerate in a tightly sealed jar for up to a week.**

Tahini Dressing

I love this dressing because it adds so much flavor for relatively few carbs. It's great on Falafel Salad (page 106) and equally delicious as a dipping sauce for a batch of Hemp Seed Nuggets (page 146).

YIELD: 5 fluid ounces (150 ml) (2 tablespoons/30 ml per serving)
PREP TIME: 3 minutes

¼ cup (64g) tahini, room temperature

Juice of 1 lemon

3 tablespoons (45 ml) water

1 teaspoon crushed garlic

In a small bowl, whisk together all the ingredients until smooth and creamy.

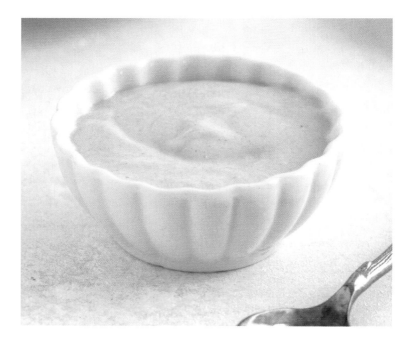

To store **Refrigerate in a tightly sealed jar for up to 5 days.**

NUTRITION INFORMATION: **76** calories | **6.4g** fat | **3g** protein | **2.4g** total carbs | **1.2g** net carbs

Keto Buttery Spread

I grew up on margarine spreads (yikes!), and though they are definitely high in fat, I wouldn't call them healthy by any means. Most of the spreads on the market are hydrogenated, and those that aren't almost always contain industrial seed oils or palm oil—not great for our bodies or the planet!

There are a few faux butters on the market that contain good-quality whole-food ingredients, but the prices are fairly prohibitive. So I decided to do a little reverse engineering on a few of my favorites, and this spread was the result! It melts just like butter and is delicious on Coconut Flour Waffles (page 60), Tahini Bagels (page 80), and toasted Seed Bread (page 74).

¾ cup (168g) refined coconut oil, softened (see Note)

¼ cup plus 2 tablespoons (90 ml) pea milk or other nondairy milk of choice

¼ cup (60 ml) extra-virgin olive oil

¼ cup (30g) roasted unsalted macadamia nuts

2 teaspoons nutritional yeast

1 teaspoon lemon juice or apple cider vinegar

¾ teaspoon salt

To store Refrigerate in a tightly sealed container for up to a week or freeze for up to 2 months.

Note I almost always use unrefined coconut oil, but this recipe is an exception. Refined coconut oil has a neutral flavor that is needed for the savory versions of this spread.

Variation GARLIC BUTTERY SPREAD. *Add 1 tablespoon of crushed garlic to the ingredients before blending, then stir in 1 tablespoon of dried parsley before chilling.*

YIELD: about 1½ cups (350 ml) (1 tablespoon per serving)
PREP TIME: 5 minutes, plus time to chill

- Put all the ingredients in a blender or food processor and blend until smooth, about 90 seconds.

- Pour into a food storage container than holds at least 1½ cups (360 ml) and refrigerate for at least 2 hours, until firm.

Variation CINNAMON BUTTERY SPREAD. *Add 1 teaspoon of ground cinnamon and 1 tablespoon of granulated sweetener to the ingredients, then blend.*

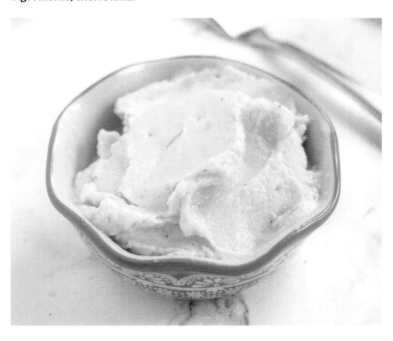

Greek Dressing

Not only is this dressing great on a Greek Salad (page 120), but it makes a pretty tasty marinade for mushrooms!

   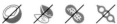

YIELD: ¾ cup (180 ml) (2 tablespoons/30 ml per serving)
PREP TIME: 3 minutes, plus 1 hour to chill

½ cup (120 ml) extra-virgin olive oil

¼ cup (60 ml) red wine vinegar

1 teaspoon dried oregano leaves

1 teaspoon crushed garlic

1 teaspoon dehydrated onion flakes

¼ tablespoon ground black pepper

In a small bowl, whisk all the ingredients together. Transfer the dressing to a tightly sealed jar or bottle and refrigerate for an hour before serving so the flavors have time to combine and the dehydrated onions to rehydrate.

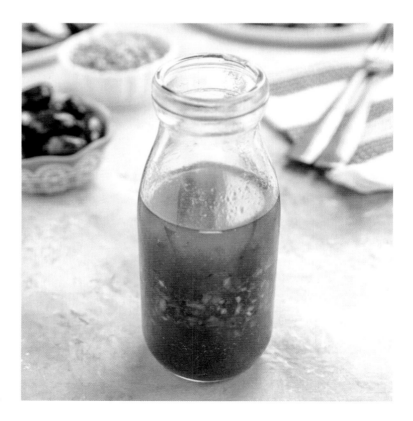

To store **Refrigerate for up to 5 days.**

Easy Vegan Pesto

Pesto is one of my favorite toppings for Zucchini Noodles (page 179), as well as my go-to pizza sauce. This pesto is not only dairy-free, but also nut-free, and it is much tastier than a jar of store-bought pesto.

  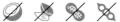

YIELD: 1⅓ cups (320 ml) (⅓ cup/80 ml per serving)
PREP TIME: 5 minutes

¾ cup (180 ml) extra-virgin olive oil

2 packed cups (60g) fresh basil leaves

¼ cup (20g) nutritional yeast

¼ cup (40g) hulled hemp seeds

1 tablespoon lemon juice

1 teaspoon crushed garlic

½ teaspoon salt

Put all the ingredients in a blender or food processor and blend until mostly smooth but not completely blended, about 90 seconds.

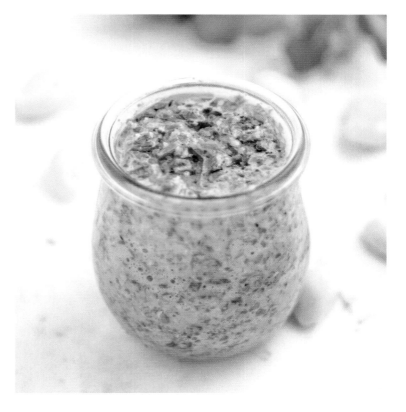

To store *Refrigerate in a tightly sealed container for up to 10 days.*

Creamy Hemp Sauce

This versatile white sauce can be used in place of Alfredo sauce, as a white pizza sauce, and pretty much anywhere you'd use a béchamel. If you have a difficult time finding hemp seeds, cashews or sunflower seeds work equally well in this recipe; just be sure to account for the difference in macros.

   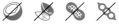

YIELD: 1⅔ cups (390 ml) (⅓ cup/about 80 ml per serving)
PREP TIME: 5 minutes

1 cup (160g) hulled hemp seeds

¾ cup (60g) nutritional yeast

¾ cup (180 ml) water

1 teaspoon crushed garlic

¼ teaspoon paprika or ground nutmeg (optional)

¼ teaspoon salt

Put all the ingredients in a blender or food processor and blend until completely smooth, 2 to 3 minutes. Pour into a pint glass or jar (475 ml) to serve.

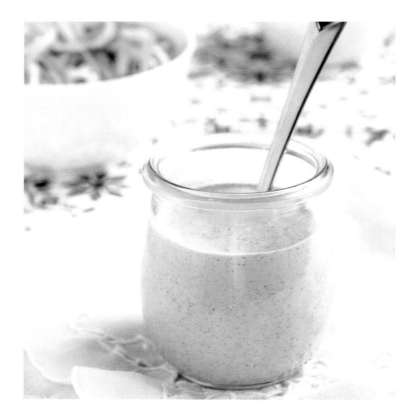

To store Refrigerate in a tightly sealed jar for up to 5 days.

NUTRITION INFORMATION: **305** calories | **20.2g** fat | **14.3g** protein | **4g** total carbs | **2.3g** net carbs

Faux Parm Sprinkles

This is basically a vegan keto version of that cheese that comes in a shaker. It's delicious on top of pizza and pesto dishes and really elevates a plate of plain roasted broccoli. But these sprinkles aren't just tasty; they pack some solid nutrition as well. Thanks to the Brazil nuts, each tablespoon of these sprinkles contains over 75 percent of the recommended daily intake of selenium, an important antioxidant and cofactor in the production of thyroid hormones.

YIELD: 1½ cups (165g) (1 tablespoon per serving)
PREP TIME: 3 minutes

½ cup (66g) raw Brazil nuts

½ cup (56g) raw macadamia nut halves

½ cup (40g) nutritional yeast

½ teaspoon salt

¼ teaspoon granulated garlic

¼ teaspoon granulated onion

Put all the ingredients in a high-powered blender or food processor and blend until the mixture has the texture of sand, 20 to 30 seconds.

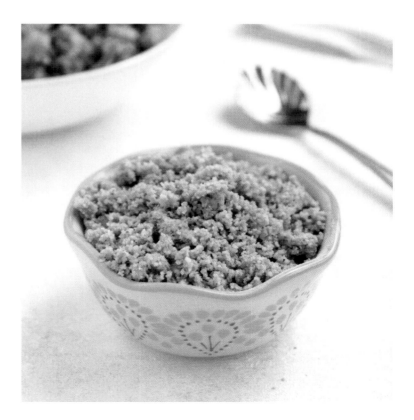

To store: Refrigerate in a tightly sealed container for up to 2 weeks.

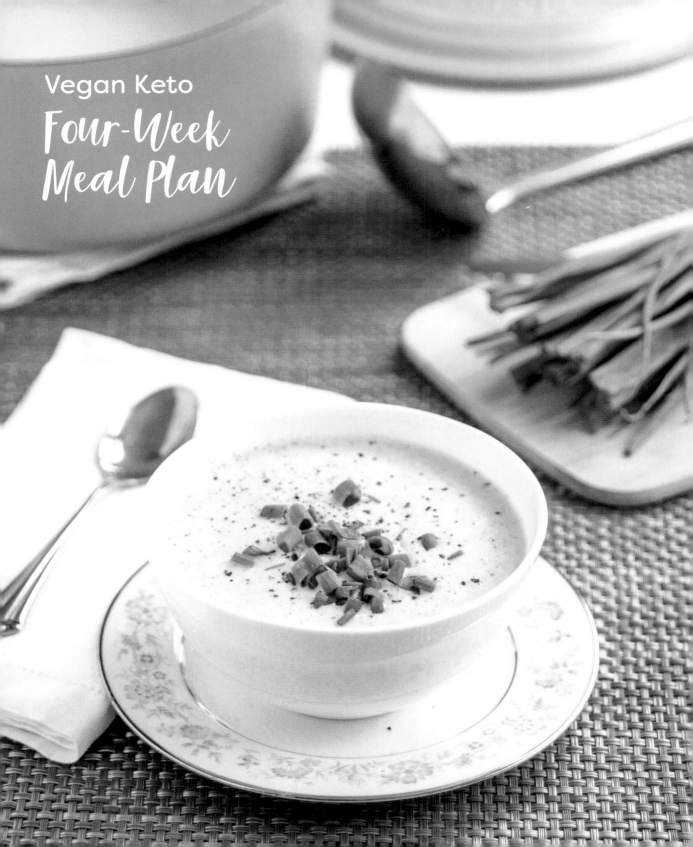

Vegan Keto
Four-Week
Meal Plan

Meal Plan *Notes*

- Weeks 1 and 2 are designed for quick entry into ketosis and provide around 20 grams of net carbs per day. Repeating the first two weeks to become fully fat-adapted is definitely an option.

- Weeks 3 and 4 offer a bit of an increase in carbohydrates for more variety in both nutrients and flavors, as well as a soy-free option for those who don't eat soy.

- Some people feel better eating more carbohydrates. If you fall into this camp, you may want to start on Week 3 of the plan and simply repeat Weeks 3 and 4.

- This plan is designed to serve one person. Be sure to double the recipes if you are serving two people.

- The plan makes generous use of leftovers. I don't have time to lock myself in the kitchen all day every day, and based on the requests you've sent me, it seems that you guys don't, either!

- The recipes that you will be making from scratch are in bold, and nonbolded recipes are leftovers. Details for preparing the italicized "mini recipes" are found in the notes for the week.

- Unless otherwise stated, the nutrition information assumes that you will eat one serving of each recipe. Where it says "x2," you should consume two servings. For two meals in Week 4, you will consume five servings of falafel.

- Most of the nonperishable ingredients are used in all four weeks, so if you buy a bag of chia seeds for use in Week 1, they will also be used in Weeks 2, 3, and 4.

- Similarly, vegetables are often used from week to week, so you may need only 1 ounce (28g) of cabbage one week but 8 ounces (225g) the next. It's not a bad idea to look ahead to the next week, compare it to the current week, and see what is already in your refrigerator or pantry!

- Produce weights are approximate.

- When you need small quantities of vegetables (1 to 2 ounces/28 to 56g), consider buying them off the salad bar to minimize waste. That way, you're not buying a whole head of cabbage when you need just a few tablespoons.

- Quantities of dry goods are rounded up slightly where necessary.

- Nuts and seeds should be purchased in raw form unless otherwise stated.

- While you can certainly make your own Keto Buttery Spread (page 187), the assumption for the shopping lists is that you will buy a vegan butter substitute.

- Salt and pepper are not included in the shopping lists, as they are most likely already in your cupboard.

- Optional ingredients (like garnishes and toppings) are not included in the shopping lists.

- You can definitely have your usual coffee or tea; just watch what you put into it. Suggestions: unsweetened nondairy milk, full-fat canned coconut milk, unsweetened nondairy creamer (check labels!), monkfruit sweetener, stevia, or erythritol-based sweetener.

- I like to drink lemon water throughout the day—1 teaspoon of lemon juice in 8 to 12 ounces (240 to 350 ml) of water. It's nice and refreshing and brings a little vitamin C and trace amounts of minerals to the game. Make sure to purchase extra lemons or lemon juice for your lemon water.

Week 1

20g
NET
CARBS

DAY 1

MEAL 1

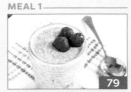

79

Almond Butter & Raspberry Chia Pudding

MEAL 2

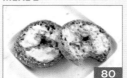

80

Tahini Bagels x2
⊕ *2 cups (56g) mixed greens*
⊕ *1 avocado, mashed*

MEAL 3

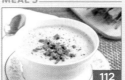

112

Creamy Cauliflower Soup
🍴 *Cooked Spinach with Pepitas & Nooch*

CALORIES:	**1560**
FAT:	**118g**
PROTEIN:	**67.7g**
TOTAL CARBS:	**78.6g**
NET CARBS:	**21.4g**

DAY 2

MEAL 1

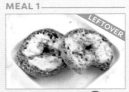
LEFTOVER

Tahini Bagels x2
⊕ *2 cups (56g) mixed greens*
⊕ *1 avocado, mashed*

MEAL 2

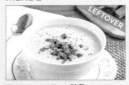
LEFTOVER

Creamy Cauliflower Soup x2

MEAL 3

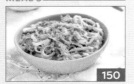

150

Zucchini Alfredo

CALORIES:	**1552**
FAT:	**114g**
PROTEIN:	**73.3g**
TOTAL CARBS:	**69.1g**
NET CARBS:	**19.4g**

DAY 3

MEAL 1

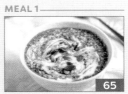

65

High-Protein "Noatmeal"

MEAL 2

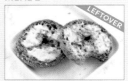
LEFTOVER

Tahini Bagels x2
⊕ *2 cups (56g) mixed greens*
⊕ *1 avocado, mashed*

MEAL 3

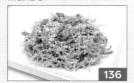

136

Kelp Noodle Pad Thai

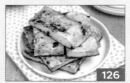

126

Chili Tamari Tofu

CALORIES:	**1507**
FAT:	**121.9g**
PROTEIN:	**67.7g**
TOTAL CARBS:	**59.4g**
NET CARBS:	**20.9g**

DAY 4

MEAL 1

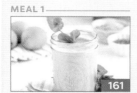
161

Rise & Shine Smoothie

MEAL 2

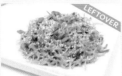

Kelp Noodle Pad Thai

MEAL 3

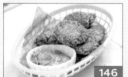
146

Hemp Seed Nuggets (x2)
👨‍🍳 *Mixed Green Salad with Pecans*

CALORIES:	**1561**
FAT:	**130.8g**
PROTEIN:	**72.2g**
TOTAL CARBS:	**54.9g**
NET CARBS:	**18.4g**

DAY 5

MEAL 1

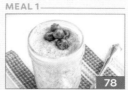
78

Basic Chia Pudding

MEAL 2

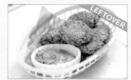

Hemp Seed Nuggets
👨‍🍳 *Mixed Green Salad with Pecans*

MEAL 3

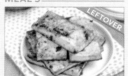

Chili Tamari Tofu (x2)
👨‍🍳 *Cooked Spinach with Pepitas & Nooch*

SNACK

➕ *¼ cup (30g) pecans*
👨‍🍳 *Celery with Mustard Vinaigrette*

CALORIES:	**1591**
FAT:	**125.2g**
PROTEIN:	**72.5g**
TOTAL CARBS:	**73.7g**
NET CARBS:	**21.5g**

DAY 6

MEAL 1

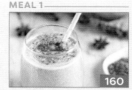
160

Golden Chai Protein Smoothie

MEAL 2

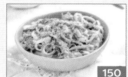

Chili Tamari Tofu   **Creamy Cauliflower Soup**

MEAL 3

150

Zucchini Alfredo
➕ *with 3 tablespoons (30g) hemp seeds*

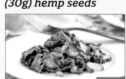
114

Warm Kale Salad

SNACK

👨‍🍳 *Celery with Mustard Vinaigrette*

CALORIES:	**1542**
FAT:	**115.9g**
PROTEIN:	**73.3g**
TOTAL CARBS:	**82.1g**
NET CARBS:	**21.5g**

DAY 7

MEAL 1

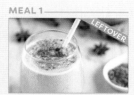

Golden Chai Protein Smoothie

MEAL 2

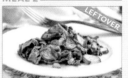

Warm Kale Salad
👨‍🍳 *Avocado with Hemp Seeds & Nooch*

MEAL 3

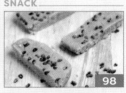
151

Buffalo Jackfruit Tacos

SNACK

98

Easy Peanut Butter Protein Bars

CALORIES:	**1577**
FAT:	**120.7g**
PROTEIN:	**79.6g**
TOTAL CARBS:	**75.8g**
NET CARBS:	**20.9g**

Week 1 Notes

MEAL PREP:

- Make the Creamy Cauliflower Soup and the bagels the day before starting the plan unless you have lots of time for cooking on Day 1.

- Make a batch of Easy Mustard Vinaigrette (page 184) for Weeks 1 and 2. If you don't like mustard, you can sub in any low-carb dressing (with 1g or fewer net carbs per serving).

DAY 1:

- **MEAL 1**
  Use frozen berries for the Almond Butter & Berry Chia Pudding.

- **MEAL 2**
  I make little sandwiches out of the bagels, greens, and mashed avocado. Split the bagels down the center, spread each half with ¼ of the mashed avocado, and stuff with the greens. You can toast the bagels beforehand if you like.

- **MEAL 3**
  🍳 Cooked Spinach with Pepitas & Nooch:
  1 cup (170g) of steamed spinach (about 5½ cups/170g of fresh baby spinach), topped with 2 tablespoons (10g) of nutritional yeast and 2 tablespoons (15g) of pepitas (pumpkin seeds).

  Freeze one serving of Creamy Cauliflower Soup for Day 6.

DAY 2:

- **MEAL 3**
  Make a half batch of the Creamy Hemp Sauce (page 190) for the Zucchini Alfredo. Use one serving today and one on Day 6.

DAY 3:

- **MEAL 3**
  You can omit the carrot from the Kelp Noodle Pad Thai unless you already have a small amount of carrot on hand.

DAY 4:

- **MEAL 3**
  🍳 Mixed Green Salad with Pecans:
  2 cups (56g) of mixed greens, 2 tablespoons (30 ml) of Easy Mustard Vinaigrette, and 3 tablespoons (23g) of chopped pecans.

DAY 5:

- **SNACK**
  🍳 Celery with Mustard Vinaigrette:
  4 stalks of celery, each about 4 inches (10 cm) long (3 ounces/85g total), dipped in 2 tablespoons (30 ml) of Easy Mustard Vinaigrette.

- Transfer the frozen portion of Creamy Cauliflower Soup to the fridge for lunch tomorrow.

DAY 6:

- **MEAL 3**
  Replace the hazelnuts in the Warm Kale Salad with pecans for ease of shopping.

DAY 7:

- **MEAL 2**
  🍳 Avocado with Hemp Seeds & Nooch:
  1 medium Hass avocado, cubed, mixed with 3 tablespoons (30g) of hulled hemp seeds and 2 tablespoons (10g) of nutritional yeast. Optional: sprinkle with chili powder. This is a frequent snack of mine.

- The remainder of the Buffalo Jackfruit Tacos and the Easy Peanut Butter Protein Bars will be consumed in Week 2.

Week 1 *Shopping List*

PRODUCE:

baby spinach, 1 pound (454g)

cauliflower, 1 medium head

celery, 8 ounces (225g)

chives, 1 tablespoon

garlic, 3 or 4 cloves

Hass avocados, 5 medium (7½ ounces/212g each)

kale, 2¼ ounces (65g)

mint, 1 or 2 sprigs

mixed greens, 10 ounces (285g)

radishes, 2 ounces (56g)

scallions, 4

zucchini, 3 small (3½ ounces/100g each)

NUTS & SEEDS:

chia seeds, 2¼ ounces (65g)

flax seeds, 7 ounces (200g)

hulled hemp seeds, 1 pound (454g)

pecans, 2¼ ounces (65g)

pepitas (pumpkin seeds), 2¼ ounces (65g)

sesame seeds, 1¼ ounces (35g)

tahini, ½ cup (128g)

unsweetened creamy almond butter, ¼ cup (64g)

unsweetened creamy peanut butter, ½ cup (128g)

FROZEN FOODS:

raspberries

REFRIGERATED ITEMS:

extra-firm tofu, 1 (14-ounce/397-g) block

nondairy milk of choice, 6 cups (1.4L)

vegan buttery spread

PANTRY ITEMS:

apple cider vinegar, 1 ounce (30 ml)

cacao nibs, 1 ounce (28g)

chili paste or Sriracha sauce, 1 tablespoon

extra-virgin olive oil, 6 ounces (180 ml)

granulated sweetener, 2 tablespoons (24g)

hot sauce, 2 ounces (60 ml)

kelp noodles, 1 (12-ounce/340-g) package

low-sodium tamari or coconut aminos, 3 tablespoons (45 ml)

nutritional yeast, 3½ ounces (100g)

pea protein powder, 4 ounces (115g)

prepared mustard of choice, 3 ounces (90 ml)

psyllium husks, 1 ounce (28g)

toasted sesame oil, 1 tablespoon

vegetable broth, 3½ cups (830 ml)

young green jackfruit in brine, 1 (17-ounce/ 482-g) can

baking powder

Chai Spice Blend (page 173)

ground cinnamon

liquid stevia

Savory Herb Blend (page 175)

turmeric powder

vanilla extract

Week 2

20g
NET
CARBS

DAY 1

MEAL 1

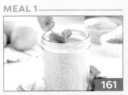
161

Rise & Shine Smoothie

MEAL 2

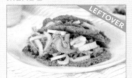
LEFTOVER

Buffalo Jackfruit Tacos
(left over from Week 1)

MEAL 3

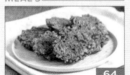
64

Sausage-Style Breakfast Patties
🍳 *Mustardy Greens*

SNACK

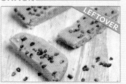
LEFTOVER

Easy Peanut Butter Protein Bars x2
(left over from Week 1)

CALORIES: **1579**
FAT: **119.5g**
PROTEIN: **72g**
TOTAL CARBS: **71.2g**
NET CARBS: **20g**

DAY 2

MEAL 1

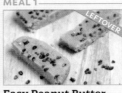
LEFTOVER

Easy Peanut Butter Protein Bars x2

MEAL 2

LEFTOVER

Sausage-Style Breakfast Patties

MEAL 3

144

Black Bean Burgers x2
🍳 *Avocado with Hemp Seeds & Nooch*

SNACK

Celery with Mustard Vinaigrette

CALORIES: **1571**
FAT: **128.9g**
PROTEIN: **77.5g**
TOTAL CARBS: **115.5g**
NET CARBS: **18.1g**

DAY 3

MEAL 1

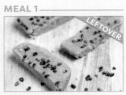
LEFTOVER

Easy Peanut Butter Protein Bars

MEAL 2

 LEFTOVER

186

Black Bean Burgers x2 ➕ *1 avocado with* **Tahini** x2 **Dressing**

MEAL 3

LEFTOVER

Sausage-Style Breakfast Patties
🍳 *Cooked Spinach with Pepitas & Nooch*

SNACK

¼ cup (30g) pecans

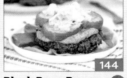

CALORIES: **1525**
FAT: **123.4g**
PROTEIN: **70.2g**
TOTAL CARBS: **52g**
NET CARBS: **19.3g**

DAY 4

MEAL 1

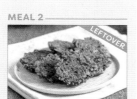

65

Overnight "Noats"

MEAL 2

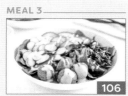

Sausage-Style Breakfast Patties

MEAL 3

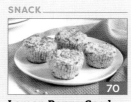

106

Falafel Salad

SNACK

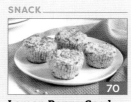

70

Lemon Poppy Seed Muffins

⊕ *1 tablespoon vegan buttery spread*

CALORIES:	**1501**
FAT:	**125.5g**
PROTEIN:	**70.4g**
TOTAL CARBS:	**46.9g**
NET CARBS:	**20g**

DAY 5

MEAL 1

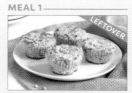

LEFTOVER

Lemon Poppy Seed Muffins x2

⊕ *2 tablespoons (28g) vegan buttery spread*

MEAL 2

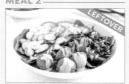

LEFTOVER

Falafel Salad

MEAL 3

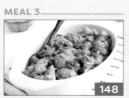

148

Cauliflower Bake

CALORIES:	**1558**
FAT:	**124.4g**
PROTEIN:	**75g**
TOTAL CARBS:	**58.9g**
NET CARBS:	**19.7g**

DAY 6

MEAL 1

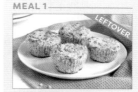

LEFTOVER

Lemon Poppy Seed Muffins x2

⊕ *2 tablespoons (28g) vegan buttery spread*

MEAL 2

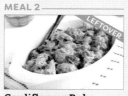

LEFTOVER

Cauliflower Bake

MEAL 3

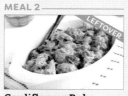

130

Sweet Chili Roasted Radishes x2

🍽 *Tahini Greens*

CALORIES:	**1531**
FAT:	**116.5g**
PROTEIN:	**83g**
TOTAL CARBS:	**57.5g**
NET CARBS:	**19.5g**

DAY 7

MEAL 1

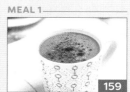

159

Keto Pumpkin Spice Latte

MEAL 2

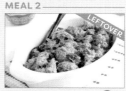

LEFTOVER

Cauliflower Bake x2

MEAL 3

SNACK

🍽 *Coconut Pecan Treat*

CALORIES:	**1556**
FAT:	**120.2g**
PROTEIN:	**72g**
TOTAL CARBS:	**73.8g**
NET CARBS:	**19.5g**

Week 2 *Notes*

DAY 1:

- **MEAL 3**

  👨‍🍳 **Mustardy Greens:** *Not to be confused with "mustard greens," this dish consists of 1 cup (170g) of steamed spinach (about 5½ cups/170g of fresh baby spinach) topped with 2 tablespoons (30 ml) of Easy Mustard Vinaigrette (which you already made for Week 1).*

DAY 3:

- **MEAL 2**

  The Tahini Dressing can go on top of the burgers, the avocado, or both.

  When making the dressing, save the zest to make the No-Cook Falafel for the Falafel Salad on Day 4 (or make them a night ahead when you make the Tahini Dressing).

DAY 6:

- **MEAL 3**

  👨‍🍳 **Tahini Greens:** *1 cup (170g) of steamed spinach (about 5½ cups/170g of fresh baby spinach) topped with 3 tablespoons (30g) of hemp seeds, 2 tablespoons (10g) of nutritional yeast, and 2 tablespoons (30 ml) of Tahini Dressing.*

  The rest of the Sweet Chili Roasted Radishes will be eaten in Week 3.

DAY 7:

- **MEAL 1**

  You can use black tea or herbal tea in place of the coffee in the Keto Pumpkin Spice Latte.

- **MEAL 2**

  The Cauliflower Bake is super filling and could easily be stretched into lunch + dinner.

- **SNACK**

  👨‍🍳 **Coconut Pecan Treat:** *I eat this a lot as a dessert or snack. It's really basic—mix ⅓ cup (80 ml) of full-fat coconut milk with ½ cup (60g) of pecans and sprinkle with cinnamon. If you don't mind the extra carbs, you can add some frozen raspberries, too.*

- Chill the remainder of the coconut milk and the pumpkin puree in preparation for Week 3!

Week 2 Shopping List

PRODUCE:

baby spinach, 1 pound plus 2 ounces (510g)

cauliflower florets, 1⅓ pounds (600g)

celery, 3 ounces (85g)

cucumber, 1 very small, or 2 Persian cucumbers (2 ounces/56g total)

garlic, 2 or 3 cloves

Hass avocado, 1 medium (7½ ounces/212g)

lemons, 2, plus 1 teaspoon juice

mint, 1 or 2 sprigs

radishes, 1 pound plus 2 ounces (510g)

red cabbage, 1 ounce (30g)

scallions, 4

NUTS & SEEDS:

chia seeds, 1½ ounces (40g)

flax seeds, 5 ounces (140g)

hulled hemp seeds, 14 ounces (400g)

pecans, 3½ ounces (100g)

pepitas (pumpkin seeds), 3 ounces (85g)

sesame seeds, 1 ounce (28g)

tahini, ½ cup (128g)

walnuts, 4½ ounces (128g)

REFRIGERATED ITEMS:

nondairy milk of choice, 2½ cups (600 ml)

vegan buttery spread

PANTRY ITEMS:

black soybeans, unsalted, 1 (15-ounce/425-g) can

chili paste or Sriracha sauce, 2 teaspoons

coconut flour, 2 ounces (56g)

coconut milk, full-fat, 1 (13½-ounce/400-ml) can

extra-virgin olive oil, ¼ cup (60 ml)

granulated sweetener, ¼ cup (48g)

low-sodium tamari or coconut aminos, 2 tablespoons (30 ml)

nutritional yeast, 3 ounces (85g)

pea protein powder, 1 ounce (28g)

prepared yellow mustard, 3 tablespoons (45 ml)

pumpkin puree, 1 (15-ounce/425-g) can

vegetable broth, ½ cup (120 ml)

baking powder

baking soda

Chai Spice Blend (page 173)

coffee

dehydrated onion flakes

dried parsley leaves

granulated garlic

granulated onion

ground cinnamon

ground cumin

liquid stevia

Sausage Spice Blend (page 172)

vanilla extract

Week 3

This plan can easily be made soy-free. Simply use coconut aminos in place of tamari in the recipes. Seriously, that's it.

DAY 1

MEAL 1
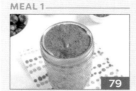
79

Silky-Smooth Chocolate Chia Pudding

MEAL 2
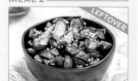

Sweet Chili Roasted Radishes (x2)
(left over from Week 2)
🍳 *Tahini Greens*

MEAL 3
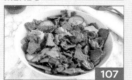
107

Fattoush Salad (x2)

SNACK
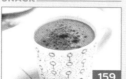
159

Iced Pumpkin Spice Latte

CALORIES:	1665
FAT:	128.8g
PROTEIN:	71.7g
TOTAL CARBS:	82.9g
NET CARBS:	25g

DAY 2

MEAL 1
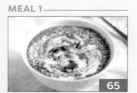
65

High-Protein "Noatmeal"

MEAL 2
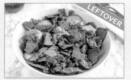
LEFTOVER

Fattoush Salad

MEAL 3
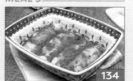
134

Cabbage Rolls
➕ *1 avocado with 2 tablespoons (10g) nutritional yeast*

SNACK
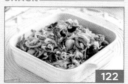
122

Mediterranean Zucchini Salad

CALORIES:	1740
FAT:	139.8g
PROTEIN:	73g
TOTAL CARBS:	77.6g
NET CARBS:	27.1g

DAY 3

MEAL 1
161

Rise & Shine Smoothie

MEAL 2

LEFTOVER LEFTOVER

Cabbage Rolls   **Mediterranean Zucchini Salad**

MEAL 3
146   129

Hemp Seed Nuggets   **Crispy Broccoli Bites** (x2)

SNACK
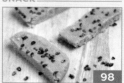
98

Easy Peanut Butter Protein Bars

CALORIES:	1662
FAT:	137.7g
PROTEIN:	74.5g
TOTAL CARBS:	62.4g
NET CARBS:	28.3g

DAY 4

MEAL 1

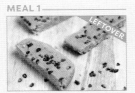
LEFTOVER

**Easy Peanut Butter
Protein Bars** (x2)

MEAL 2

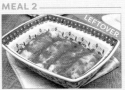
LEFTOVER

Cabbage Rolls (x2)

MEAL 3

LEFTOVER   LEFTOVER

**Hemp
Seed
Nuggets**   **Crispy
Broccoli
Bites** (x2)

CALORIES: **1527**
FAT: **125.9g**
PROTEIN: **70.9g**
TOTAL CARBS: **61.8g**
NET CARBS: **27.6g**

DAY 5

MEAL 1

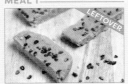
LEFTOVER

**Easy Peanut Butter
Protein Bars** (x2)

MEAL 2

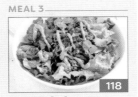
LEFTOVER   LEFTOVER

**Mediterranean
Zucchini
Salad** (x2)   **Hemp
Seed
Nuggets**

MEAL 3

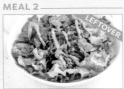
118

Taco Salad

SNACK

🍳 *Coconut Pecan
Treat (½ serving)*

CALORIES: **1616**
FAT: **134.1g**
PROTEIN: **73.4g**
TOTAL CARBS: **63.4g**
NET CARBS: **29.2g**

DAY 6

MEAL 1

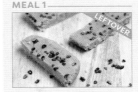
LEFTOVER

**Easy Peanut Butter
Protein Bars**
🍳 *Coconut Pecan
Treat (½ serving)*

MEAL 2

LEFTOVER

Taco Salad

MEAL 3

🍳 *Salsa Avocado*

SNACK

160

**Golden Chai Protein
Smoothie**

CALORIES: **1648**
FAT: **137.2g**
PROTEIN: **72.3g**
TOTAL CARBS: **59.9g**
NET CARBS: **22.3g**

DAY 7

MEAL 1

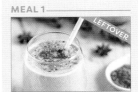
LEFTOVER

**Golden Chai Protein
Smoothie**

MEAL 2

🍳 *Salsa Avocado*

MEAL 3

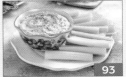
140   121

**Korean
BBQ Tacos**   **Garlic
Ginger
Slaw** (x2)

SNACK

93

Lupini Hummus (x2)
➕ *1 cup (100g)
cucumber slices*

CALORIES: **1691**
FAT: **136.9g**
PROTEIN: **70.7g**
TOTAL CARBS: **73.3g**
NET CARBS: **29.5g**

Week 3 *Notes*

- This plan can easily be made soy-free. Simply use coconut aminos in place of tamari in the recipes. Seriously, that's it.

- If you are starting with Week 3 without having followed Weeks 1 and 2, ignore the "From Previous Shopping Lists" section in the shopping list and purchase the additional items listed under "If Starting with Week 3 as the First Week."

DAY 1:

- **MEAL 1**

  Freeze the remainder of the pumpkin puree in an ice cube tray in 2-tablespoon (32-g) portions for future pumpkin lattes.

  Freeze the remainder of the coconut milk for later in the week.

- **MEAL 2**

  🍴 **Tahini Greens:** *1 cup (170g) of steamed spinach (about 5½ cups/170g of fresh baby spinach) topped with 2 tablespoons (30 ml) of Tahini Dressing.*

  If you are starting with Week 3 as your first week, make a half batch of Sweet Chili Roasted Radishes (page 130).

DAY 4:

- Transfer the frozen coconut milk to the fridge to thaw for tomorrow (or do it on the morning of Day 5).

DAY 5:

- **MEAL 2**

  Omit the Tangy Avocado Mayo from the Taco Salad.

- **SNACK**

  🍴 **Coconut Pecan Treat:** *I eat this a lot as a dessert or snack. It's really basic—mix ⅓ cup (80 ml) of full-fat coconut milk with ½ cup (60g) of pecans and sprinkle with cinnamon. If you don't mind the extra carbs, you can add some frozen raspberries, too.* You can either make the entire batch at once, split it into two servings, and chill one serving overnight, or just make a half serving at a time.

DAY 6:

- **MEAL 2**

  🍴 **Salsa Avocado:** *1 medium Hass avocado, cubed, topped with 2 tablespoons (20g) of hemp seeds, 2 tablespoons (10g) of nutritional yeast, and 2 tablespoons (32g) of salsa.*

DAY 7:

- **MEAL 3**

  Omit the Tangy Avocado Mayo from the Korean BBQ Tacos.

- The remainder of the Korean BBQ Tacos, Garlic Ginger Slaw, and Lupini Hummus are included in the Week 4 plan.

Week 3 shopping list

PRODUCE:

baby spinach, 8 ounces (225g)

broccoli florets, 8 ounces (225g)

carrots, 1 ounce (28g) shredded

cauliflower, riced, 3 ounces (85g)

cherry tomatoes, 4 ounces (115g)

cucumber, 1 medium
(7 ounces/200g)

garlic, 6 or 7 cloves

ginger, 1-inch (2.5-cm) knob

green cabbage, 1 medium head
(4 inches/10 cm in diameter—
you want larger leaves for the
Cabbage Rolls)

Hass avocados, 4 medium
(7½ ounces/212g each)

lemons, 3, or 4 ounces (120 ml)
lemon juice

mint, 1 bunch

mixed greens, 4 ounces (115g)

onion, 1 very small (2 inches/
5 cm in diameter)

parsley, 1 bunch

red cabbage, 1 small head
(4 inches/10 cm in diameter)

romaine hearts, 2 large
(7 ounces/200g)

scallions, 7 to 8

zucchini, 1 medium (7 ounces/
200g)

NUTS & SEEDS:

chia seeds, 1¼ ounces (35g)

flax seeds, 10 ounces (285g)

hulled hemp seeds, 14 ounces
(400g)

sesame seeds, 1 ounce (28g)

sunflower seeds, 1¼ ounces
(35g)

tahini, ½ cup (64g)

walnuts, 8½ ounces (240g)

REFRIGERATED ITEMS:

nondairy milk of choice,
40 ounces (1.2L)

salsa, 4 ounces (120 ml)

PANTRY ITEMS:

cacao nibs, ¼ cup (30g)

chili paste, 1 teaspoon

cocoa powder, 1 tablespoon

extra-virgin olive oil, 8 ounces
(240 ml)

granulated sweetener,
2 tablespoons (24g)

low-sodium tamari or
coconut aminos, 3½ ounces
(105 ml)

lupini beans, in brine,
1 (12-ounce/340-g) jar

nutritional yeast, 2½ ounces
(70g)

pea protein powder,
4½ ounces (128g)

psyllium husks, 2 tablespoons
(10g)

sun-dried tomatoes,
3 or 4 pieces (10g)

toasted sesame oil, 1 ounce
(30 ml)

tomato sauce, low-sugar,
1 (24-ounce/710-ml) jar or can

unseasoned rice wine vinegar,
1 tablespoon

unsweetened creamy peanut
butter, ½ cup (128g)

vegetable broth, 6 ounces
(180 ml)

baking powder

Chai Spice Blend (page 173)

chili powder

coffee

dried oregano leaves

dried parsley leaves

granulated garlic

ground cinnamon

ground cumin

liquid stevia

paprika

Savory Herb Blend (page 175)

turmeric powder

vanilla extract

za'atar seasoning

**FROM PREVIOUS
SHOPPING LISTS:**

coconut milk, full-fat canned,
²/₃ cup (160 ml)

pumpkin puree, 2 tablespoons
(30g)

**IF STARTING WITH WEEK 3
AS THE FIRST WEEK:**

chili paste, 1 teaspoon

coconut milk, full-fat,
1 (13½-ounce/400-ml) can

extra-virgin olive oil,
1 tablespoon

granulated sweetener,
1 teaspoon

low-sodium tamari or
coconut aminos, 1 tablespoon

pumpkin puree, 1 (15-ounce/
425-g) can

radishes, 8 ounces (225g)

scallion, 1

sesame seeds, 1 teaspoon

Week 4

This plan can easily be made soy-free. Simply use coconut aminos in place of tamari in the recipes. Seriously, that's it.

DAY 1

MEAL 1

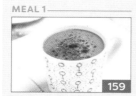
`159`

Iced Pumpkin Spice Latte

MEAL 2

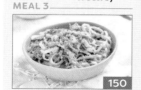

Korean BBQ Tacos (left over from Week 3)

Garlic Ginger `x2` **Slaw** (left over from Week 3)

MEAL 3

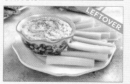
`150`

Zucchini Alfredo
➕ *1 tablespoon nutritional yeast*

SNACK

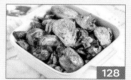

Lupini Hummus `x2` (left over from Week 3)
➕ *1 cup (100g) cucumber slices*

CALORIES: **1627**
FAT: **127g**
PROTEIN: **71.9g**
TOTAL CARBS: **82.9g**
NET CARBS: **25g**

DAY 2

MEAL 1

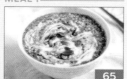
`65`

Overnight "Noats"

MEAL 2

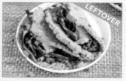

Korean BBQ Tacos

MEAL 3

🍳 *Spinach Marinara*
➕ *¼ cup (40g) hemp seeds*

SNACK

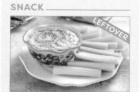

Lupini Hummus `x2`
➕ *1 cup (120g) radish slices*

CALORIES: **1652**
FAT: **135.5g**
PROTEIN: **73g**
TOTAL CARBS: **62.1g**
NET CARBS: **24.7g**

DAY 3

MEAL 1

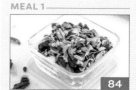
`84`

Coco-Nutty Trail Mix `x2`
➕ *1 cup (240 ml) nondairy milk*

MEAL 2

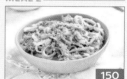
`150`

Zucchini Alfredo
➕ *1 tablespoon nutritional yeast*

MEAL 3

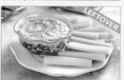
`128`

Tangy Brussels Sprouts `x2` **with Walnuts & Mushrooms**
➕ *1 tablespoon nutritional yeast*

SNACK

Lupini Hummus `x2`
➕ *1 cup (120g) radish slices*
➕ *¼ cup (28g) pepitas (pumpkin seeds)*

CALORIES: **1641**
FAT: **131.5g**
PROTEIN: **72.3g**
TOTAL CARBS: **62.4g**
NET CARBS: **29.8g**

DAY 4

MEAL 1

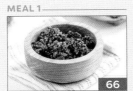

66

Nut-Free Chocolate Granola (x2)

⊕ *1 cup (240 ml) nondairy milk*

MEAL 2

114

Tangy Brussels Sprouts with Walnuts & Mushrooms

Warm Kale Salad

MEAL 3

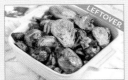

Tangy Brussels Sprouts with Walnuts & Mushrooms

👨‍🍳 *Spinach Marinara*

⊕ *¼ cup (40g) hemp seeds*

SNACK

Lupini (x2) **Hummus**

Coco-Nutty Trail Mix

⊕ *1 cup (120g) radish slices*

CALORIES: **1712**
FAT: **147.2g**
PROTEIN: **71.4g**
TOTAL CARBS: **66.7g**
NET CARBS: **26.7g**

DAY 5

MEAL 1

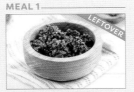

Nut-Free Chocolate Granola (x2)

⊕ *1 cup (240 ml) nondairy milk*

MEAL 2

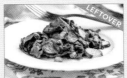

Warm Kale Salad

MEAL 3

88

186

No-Cook Falafel (x5)

Tahini Dressing (x2)

SNACK

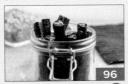

96

Nori Energy Sticks (x2)

CALORIES: **1737**
FAT: **152.5g**
PROTEIN: **71.9g**
TOTAL CARBS: **58g**
NET CARBS: **22.6g**

DAY 6

MEAL 1

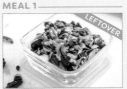

Coco-Nutty Trail Mix (x2)

⊕ *1 cup (240 ml) nondairy milk*

MEAL 2

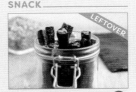

No-Cook Falafel (x5)

Tahini Dressing (x2)

MEAL 3

👨‍🍳 *Spinach Marinara*

SNACK

Nori Energy Sticks (x2)

CALORIES: **1680**
FAT: **139.6g**
PROTEIN: **73.5g**
TOTAL CARBS: **65g**
NET CARBS: **27.4g**

DAY 7

MEAL 1

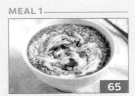

65

High-Protein "Noatmeal"

MEAL 2

Nori Energy Sticks (x2)

MEAL 3

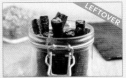

100

Cucumber Avocado Pinwheels (x2)

Tahini Dressing

SNACK

Coco-Nutty Trail Mix

Nut-Free Chocolate Granola

CALORIES: **1624**
FAT: **135.4g**
PROTEIN: **71.5g**
TOTAL CARBS: **72.5g**
NET CARBS: **20.4g**

Week 4 *Notes*

- **MEAL 1**
  This latte will finish up the can of coconut milk.

  You will still have plenty of pumpkin cubes in the freezer for future use!

- **MEAL 3**
  Make a half batch of the Creamy Hemp Sauce (page 190) for the Zucchini Alfredo. Use one serving today and one on Day 3.

DAY 2: _____

- **MEAL 3**
  🍴 Spinach Marinara: *1 cup (170g) of steamed spinach (about 5½ cups/170g of fresh baby spinach) topped with ½ cup (120 ml) of tomato sauce, 2 tablespoons (10g) of nutritional yeast, and ¼ cup (40g) of hulled hemp seeds.*

  Remember, you should have leftover tomato sauce in the fridge from the Cabbage Rolls in Week 3!

- To save time in the morning on Day 3, make the Zucchini Alfredo tonight.

DAY 3: _____

- **MEAL 1**
  I like to eat this trail mix like cereal sometimes—pour it into a large cereal bowl, cover with the nondairy milk, and dive in.

DAY 4: _____

- **MEAL 2**
  Replace the hazelnuts in the Warm Kale Salad with pecans for ease of shopping.

- Make the Nori Energy Sticks tonight and pop them in your lunch box in the a.m.

Week 4 Shopping List

PRODUCE:

baby spinach, 1¼ pounds (570g)

broccoli sprouts, 1¼ ounces (35g)

Brussels sprouts, 8½ ounces (240g)

cremini mushrooms, 7 ounces (200g)

cucumber, 1 small (5½ ounces/155g)

garlic, 2 or 3 cloves

Hass avocado, 1 medium (7½ ounces/212g each)

kale, 4 cups chopped (2¼ ounces/65g)

lemon, 1

radishes, 15 ounces (420g)

zucchini, 3 small (3½ ounces/100g each)

NUTS & SEEDS:

chia seeds, 1 ounce (28g)

flax seeds, 1 ounce (28g)

hulled hemp seeds, 1 pound plus 1 ounce (480g)

pecans, 5½ ounces (155g)

pepitas (pumpkin seeds), 5½ ounces (155g)

sesame seeds, 2 ounces (56g)

sunflower seeds, 4½ ounces (128g)

tahini, 4½ ounces (80g)

walnuts, 1¼ ounces (35g)

REFRIGERATED ITEMS:

nondairy milk of choice, 44 ounces (1.3L)

PANTRY ITEMS:

apple cider vinegar, 1 tablespoon

cacao nibs, 1¼ ounces (35g)

cocoa powder, 2 tablespoons (20g)

extra-virgin olive oil, 2 ounces (60 ml)

granulated sweetener, 2 tablespoons (24g)

nutritional yeast, 2¾ ounces (78g)

pea protein powder, 1 ounce (28g)

prepared mustard of choice, 3 tablespoons (45 ml)

sushi nori, 6 sheets

unsweetened coconut flakes, 2¼ ounces (65g)

chili powder

coffee

dried parsley leaves

granulated garlic

granulated onion

ground cinnamon

ground cumin

liquid stevia

vanilla extract

FROM PREVIOUS SHOPPING LISTS:

coconut milk, full-fat, ⅓ cup (80 ml)

pumpkin puree, 2 tablespoons (30g)

tomato sauce, low-sugar, 1½ cups (350 ml)

References

1 Dimitriadis, G., Mitrou, P., Lambadiari, V., Maratou, E., and Raptis, S. "Insulin Effects in Muscle and Adipose Tissue." *Diabetes Research and Clinical Practice* 93 (2011): S52–S59.

2 Schaefer, E. J., Gleason, J. A., and Dansinger, M. L. "Dietary Fructose and Glucose Differentially Affect Lipid and Glucose Homeostasis." *Journal of Nutrition* 139, no. 6 (2009): 1257S–1262S.

3 Hassan, K. "Nonalcoholic Fatty Liver Disease: A Comprehensive Review of a Growing Epidemic." *World Journal of Gastroenterology* 20, no. 34 (2014): 12082.

4 Penckofer, S., Quinn, L., Byrn, M., Ferrans, C., Miller, M., and Strange, P. "Does Glycemic Variability Impact Mood and Quality of Life?" *Diabetes Technology & Therapeutics* 14, no. 4 (2012): 303–310.

5 Ibid.

6 Stanhope, K. L. "Sugar Consumption, Metabolic Disease and Obesity: The State of the Controversy." *Critical Reviews in Clinical Laboratory Sciences* 53, no. 1 (2016): 52–67.

7 Yancy, W. S., Foy, M., Chalecki, A. M., Vernon, M. C., and Westman, E. C. "A Low-Carbohydrate, Ketogenic Diet to Treat Type 2 Diabetes." *Nutrition & Metabolism* 2 (2005): 34.

8 "Diabetic Ketoacidosis (DKA)." U.S. National Library of Medicine (2018). Available at www.ncbi.nlm.nih.gov/pubmedhealth/PMHT0024412/

9 Paoli, A. "Ketogenic Diet for Obesity: Friend or Foe?" *International Journal of Environmental Research and Public Health* 11, no. 2 (2014): 2092–2107.

10 Davis, C., Bryan, J., Hodgson, J., and Murphy, K. "Definition of the Mediterranean Diet: A Literature Review." *Nutrients* 7, no. 11 (2015): 9139–53.

11 Chen, Z. Y., Ratnayake, W. M. N., and Cunnane, S. C. "Oxidative Stability of Flaxseed Lipids During Baking." *Journal of American Oil Chemists' Society* 71 (1994): 629.

12 Sarter, B., Kelsey, K., Schwartz, T., and Harris, W. "Blood Docosahexaenoic Acid and Eicosapentaenoic Acid in Vegans: Associations with Age and Gender and Effects of an Algal-Derived Omega-3 Fatty Acid Supplement." *Clinical Nutrition* 34, no. 2 (2015): 212–218. Available at www.clinicalnutritionjournal.com/article/S0261-5614(14)00076-4/fulltext. Accessed June 14, 2018. It's also worth noting here that omnivores tend to have low baseline levels of omega-3 fatty acids.

13 Ibid.

14 "Inflammation: A Unifying Theory of Disease." *Harvard Health Letter.* Harvard Health Publishing (2006). Available at www.health.harvard.edu/newsletter_article/Inflammation_A_unifying_theory_of_disease. Accessed June 16, 2018.

15 Simopoulos, A. P. "An Increase in the Omega-6/Omega-3 Fatty Acid Ratio Increases the Risk for Obesity." *Nutrients* 8, no. 3 (2016): 128.

16 Ibid.

17 Ibid.

18 Gibson, R., Muhlhausler, B., and Makrides, M. "Conversion of Linoleic Acid and Alpha-Linolenic Acid to Long-Chain Polyunsaturated Fatty Acids (LCPUFAs), with a Focus on Pregnancy, Lactation and the First 2 Years of Life." *Maternal & Child Nutrition* 7 (2011): 17–26.

19 Ibid.

20 Conquer, J. A., and Holub, B. J. "Supplementation with an Algae Source of Docosahexaenoic Acid Increases (n-3) Fatty Acid Status and Alters Selected Risk Factors for Heart Disease in Vegetarian Subjects." *Journal of Nutrition* 12, no. 126 (1996): 3032–39.

21 Nutrient Data Laboratory (U.S.) and Consumer and Food Economics Institute (U.S.) (1999). USDA Nutrient Database for Standard Reference. Riverdale, Maryland: USDA, Nutrient Data Laboratory, Agricultural Research Service.

22 De Souza, R. J., Mente, A., Maroleanu, A., Cozma, A. I., Ha, V., Kishibe, T., Uleryk, E., et al. "Intake of Saturated and Trans Unsaturated Fatty Acids and Risk of All Cause Mortality, Cardiovascular Disease, and Type 2 Diabetes: Systematic Review and Meta-Analysis of Observational Studies." *British Medical Journal* 351 (2015): h3978.

23 Brownell, K., and Pomeranz, J. "The Trans-Fat Ban—Food Regulation and Long-Term Health." *New England Journal of Medicine* 370, no. 19 (2014): 1773–75.

24 "Position of the American Dietetic Association: Vegetarian Diets." *Journal of the American Dietetic Association* 109, no. 7 (2009): 1266–82.

25 De Gavelle, E., Huneau, J.-F., Bianchi, C. M., Verger, E. O., and Mariotti, F. "Protein Adequacy Is Primarily a Matter of Protein Quantity, Not Quality: Modeling an Increase in Plant:Animal Protein Ratio in French Adults." *Nutrients* 9, no. 12 (2017): 1333.

26 Schaafsma, G. "The Protein Digestibility–Corrected Amino Acid Score." *Journal of Nutrition* 7, no. 130 (2000): 1865S–1867S.

27 Rogerson, D. "Vegan Diets: Practical Advice for Athletes and Exercisers." *Journal of the International Society of Sports Nutrition* 14 (2017): 36.

28 de Jager, J., Kooy, A., Lehert, P., Wulffelé, M. G., van der Kolk, J., Bets, D., Verburg, J., et al. "Long Term Treatment with Metformin in Patients with Type 2 Diabetes and Risk of Vitamin B-12 Deficiency: Randomised Placebo Controlled Trial." *British Medical Journal* 340 (2010): c2181.

29 Watanabe, F., Yabuta, Y., Bito, T., and Teng, F. "Vitamin B12-Containing Plant Food Sources for Vegetarians." *Nutrients* 6, no. 5 (2014): 1861–73.

30 Rizzo, G., Laganà, A. S., Rapisarda, A. M. C., La Ferrera, G. M. G., Buscema, M., Rossetti, P., Nigro, A., et al. "Vitamin B12 Among Vegetarians: Status, Assessment and Supplementation." *Nutrients* 8, no. 12 (2016): 767.

31 Herbert, V. "Vitamin B12." In *Present Knowledge in Nutrition,* 17th ed. Washington, D.C.: International Life Sciences Institute Press, 1996.

32 "Pantothenic Acid: Fact Sheet for Health Professionals." Office of Dietary Supplements, National Institutes of Health (2018). Available at https://ods.od.nih.gov/factsheets/PantothenicAcid-HealthProfessional/

33 "Vitamin C: Fact Sheet for Health Professionals." Office of Dietary Supplements, National Institutes of Health (2018). Available at https://ods.od.nih.gov/factsheets/VitaminC-HealthProfessional/

34 Ibid.

35 Ho-Pham, L. T., Vu, B. Q., Lai, T. Q., Nguyen, N. D., and Nguyen, T. V. "Vegetarianism, Bone Loss, Fracture and Vitamin D: A Longitudinal Study in Asian Vegans and Non-Vegans." *European Journal of Clinical Nutrition* 66 (2012): 75–82.

36 Elorinne, A.-L., Alfthan, G., Erlund, I., Kivimäki, H., Paju, A., Salminen, I., Turpeinen, U., et al. "Food and Nutrient Intake and Nutritional Status of Finnish Vegans and Non-Vegetarians." *PLoS ONE* 11, no. 2 (2016): e0148235.

37 Norman, Anthony W. "From Vitamin D to Hormone D: Fundamentals of the Vitamin D Endocrine System Essential for Good Health." *American Journal of Clinical Nutrition* 2, no. 88 (2008): 491S–499S.

38 Ibid.

39 Keegan, R.-J. H., Lu, Z., Bogusz, J. M., Williams, J. E., and Holick, M. F. "Photobiology of Vitamin D in Mushrooms and Its Bioavailability in Humans." *Dermato-Endocrinology* 5, no. 1 (2013): 165–176.

40 Jäpelt, R. B., and Jakobsen, J. "Vitamin D in Plants: A Review of Occurrence, Analysis, and Biosynthesis." *Frontiers in Plant Science* 4 (2013): 136.

41 Dyett, P., Rajaram, S., Haddad, E. H., and Sabate, J. "Evaluation of a Validated Food Frequency Questionnaire for Self-Defined Vegans in the United States." *Nutrients* 6, no. 7 (2014): 2523–39.

42 "Calcium: Fact Sheet for Consumers." Office of Dietary Supplements, National Institutes of Health (2018). Available at https://ods.od.nih.gov/Factsheets/Calcium/. Accessed June 13, 2018.

43 "Iodine: Fact Sheet for Health Professionals." Office of Dietary Supplements, National Institutes of Health (2018). Available at https://ods.od.nih.gov/factsheets/Iodine-HealthProfessional/

44 Rogerson, 2017.

45 "Iron: Fact Sheet for Health Professionals." Office of Dietary Supplements, National Institutes of Health (2018). Available at https://ods.od.nih.gov/factsheets/Iron-HealthProfessional/

46 Rogerson, 2017.

47 "Magnesium: Fact Sheet for Health Professionals." Office of Dietary Supplements, National Institutes of Health (2018). Available at https://ods.od.nih.gov/factsheets/Magnesium-HealthProfessional/

48 "Potassium: Fact Sheet for Health Professionals." Office of Dietary Supplements, National Institutes of Health (2018). Available at https://ods.od.nih.gov/factsheets/Potassium-HealthProfessional/. Accessed June 15, 2018.

49 Ibid.

50 "Zinc: Fact Sheet for Health Professionals." Office of Dietary Supplements, National Institutes of Health (2018). Available at https://ods.od.nih.gov/factsheets/Zinc-HealthProfessional/. Accessed June 12, 2018.

51 Rogerson, 2017.

52 Gupta, L., Khandelwal, D., Kalra, S., Gupta, P., Dutta, D., and Aggarwal, S. "Ketogenic Diet in Endocrine Disorders: Current Perspectives." *Journal of Postgraduate Medicine* 63, no. 4 (2017): 242–251.

53 Ibid.

54 Masino, S. A., and Ruskin, D. N. "Ketogenic Diets and Pain." *Journal of Child Neurology* 28, no. 8 (2013): 993–1001.

55 Miller, V. J., Villamena, F. A., and Volek, J. S. "Nutritional Ketosis and Mitohormesis: Potential Implications for Mitochondrial Function and Human Health." *Journal of Nutrition and Metabolism* (2018): 5157645.

56 Rizzo, G., and Baroni, L. "Soy, Soy Foods and Their Role in Vegetarian Diets." *Nutrients* 10, no. 1 (2018): 43.

57 Ibid.

58 Sarter, B., Kelsey, K., Schwartz, T., and Harris, W. "Blood Docosahexaenoic Acid and Eicosapentaenoic Acid in Vegans: Associations with Age and Gender and Effects of an Algal-Derived Omega-3 Fatty Acid Supplement." *Clinical Nutrition* 34, no. 2 (2015): 212–218. Available at www.clinicalnutritionjournal.com/article/S0261-5614(14)00076-4/fulltext. Accessed June 14, 2018.

59 Zajac, A., Poprzecki, S., Maszczyk, A., Czuba, M., Michalczyk, M., and Zydek, G. "The Effects of a Ketogenic Diet on Exercise Metabolism and Physical Performance in Off-Road Cyclists." *Nutrients* 6, no. 7 (2014): 2493–2508.

60 Trexler, E. T., Smith-Ryan, A. E., and Norton, L. E. "Metabolic Adaptation to Weight Loss: Implications for the Athlete." *Journal of the International Society of Sports Nutrition* 11, no. 7 (2014): 7.

61 Watanabe, S., Hirakawa, A., Utada, I., et al. "Ketone Body Production and Excretion During Wellness Fasting." *Diabetes Research Open Journal* 3, no. 1 (2017): 1–8.

62 National Research Council (U.S.) Subcommittee on the Tenth Edition of the Recommended Dietary Allowances. "Water and Electrolytes." In *Recommended Dietary Allowances*, 10th Edition. Washington, D.C.: National Academies Press, 1989. Available from: www.ncbi.nlm.nih.gov/books/NBK234935/

63 Miller, K. C. "Electrolyte and Plasma Responses After Pickle Juice, Mustard, and Deionized Water Ingestion in Dehydrated Humans." *Journal of Athletic Training* 49, no. 3 (2014): 360–367.

64 Schulte, E. M., Smeal, J. K., and Gearhardt, A. N. "Foods Are Differentially Associated with Subjective Effect Report Questions of Abuse Liability." *PLoS ONE* 12, no. 8 (2017): e0184220.

65 Liu, R. H. "Health Benefits of Fruit and Vegetables Are from Additive and Synergistic Combinations of Phytochemicals." *American Journal of Clinical Nutrition* 3, no. 78 (2003): 517S–520S.

66 Ibid.

67 Parvez, S., Malik, K., Ah Kang, S., and Kim, H. "Probiotics and Their Fermented Food Products Are Beneficial for Health." *Journal of Applied Microbiology* 100, no. 6 (2006): 1171–85.

68 Ibid.

69 Steenbergen, L., Sellaro, R., van Hemert, S., Bosch, J., and Colzato, L. "A Randomized Controlled Trial to Test the Effect of Multispecies Probiotics on Cognitive Reactivity to Sad Mood." *Brain, Behavior, and Immunity* 48 (2015): 258–264.

70 LeBlanc, J., Laiño, J., del Valle, M., Vannini, V., van Sinderen, D., Taranto, M., et al. "B-Group Vitamin Production by Lactic Acid Bacteria—Current Knowledge and Potential Applications." *Journal of Applied Microbiology* 111, no. 6 (2011): 1297–1309.

Recipe Index

Breakfast

 60
Coconut Flour Waffles

 62
Spinach & Olive Mini Quiche Cups

 64
Sausage-Style Breakfast Patties

 65
High-Protein "Noatmeal"

 66
Nut-Free Chocolate Granola

 68
Coconut Yogurt

 70
Lemon Poppy Seed Muffins

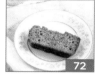 72
Pumpkin Bread

 74
Seed Bread

 76
Avocado Toast

 78
Chia Pudding Three Ways

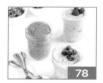 80
Tahini Bagels

Snacks

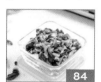 84
Coco-Nutty Trail Mix

 86
Baked Radish Chips

 88
No-Cook Falafel

 90
Flaxitos

 92
Garlic Dill Kale Chips

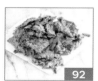 93
Lupini Hummus

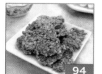 94
Seed Crackers

 96
Nori Energy Sticks

 98
Easy Peanut Butter Protein Bars

 100
Cucumber Avocado Pinwheels

 102
Curry Tofu Salad Bites

Soups, Salads & Sides

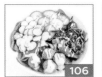
Falafel Salad
106

Fattoush Salad
107

Carrot Ginger Soup
108

Spicy Coconut Soup
110

Creamy Cauliflower Soup
112

Warm Kale Salad
114

Portabella and Summer Squash Salad
115

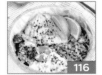
Green Keto Balance Bowl
116

Taco Salad
118

Greek Salad
120

Garlic Ginger Slaw
121

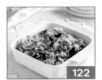
Mediterranean Zucchini Salad
122

Lemon Pesto Greens
123

Cucumber Salad
124

Chili Tamari Tofu
126

Tangy Brussels Sprouts with Mushrooms & Walnuts
128

Crispy Broccoli Bites
129

Sweet Chili Roasted Radishes
130

Main Courses

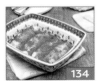
Cabbage Rolls
134

Kelp Noodle Pad Thai
136

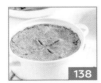
Keto Pot Pie
138

Korean BBQ Tacos
140

Meal Prep Chili
142

Smashed Bean Sandwiches
143

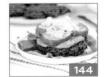
Black Bean Burgers
144

Hemp Seed Nuggets
146

Cauliflower Bake
148

Zucchini Bolognese
149

Zucchini Alfredo
150

Buffalo Jackfruit Tacos
151

Drinks & Desserts

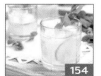 154 Sparkling Ginger Limeade

 156 Blackberry Lemonade

 158 Coconut Matcha Latte

 159 Keto Pumpkin Spice Latte

 160 Golden Chai Protein Smoothie

 161 Rise & Shine Smoothie

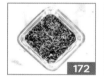 162 Chocolate Almond Butter Cupcakes

 164 Keto Black Bean Brownies

 166 Chocolate Keto Nice Cream

 168 Snickerdoodles

Basics

 172 Sausage Spice Blend

 173 Chai Spice Blend

 174 Everything Bagel Blend

 175 Savory Herb Blend

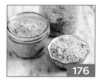 176 Nut & Seed Flours

 178 Cauliflower Rice

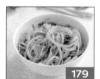 179 Zucchini Noodles

 180 Flax Tortillas

 182 Flax Egg

 183 Tangy Avocado Mayo

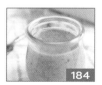 184 Easy Mustard Vinaigrette

 185 Quick Hemp Seed Sour Cream

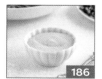 186 Tahini Dressing

 187 Keto Buttery Spread

 188 Greek Dressing

 189 Easy Vegan Pesto

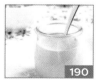 190 Creamy Hemp Sauce

 191 Faux Parm Sprinkles

Recipe Quick Reference

RECIPES	PAGE	🥥	🥜	🥜	🫘
Coconut Flour Waffles	60		✓	✓	✓
Spinach & Olive Mini Quiche Cups	62	✓	✓	✓	
Sausage-Style Breakfast Patties	64	✓		✓	✓
High-Protein "Noatmeal"	65		✓	✓	✓
Nut-Free Chocolate Granola	66	✓	✓	✓	✓
Coconut Yogurt	68		✓	✓	✓
Lemon Poppy Seed Muffins	70		✓	✓	✓
Pumpkin Bread	72		✓	✓	
Seed Bread	74	✓	✓	✓	✓
Avocado Toast	76	✓	✓	✓	✓
Basic Chia Pudding	78		✓	✓	✓
Almond Butter & Raspberry Chia Pudding	79	✓		✓	✓
Silky Smooth Chocolate Chia Pudding	79		✓	✓	✓
Tahini Bagels	80	✓	✓	✓	✓
Coco-Nutty Trail Mix	84		✓	✓	✓
Baked Radish Chips	86	✓	✓	✓	✓
No-Cook Falafel	88	✓	✓	✓	✓
Flaxitos	90	✓	✓	✓	✓
Garlic Dill Kale Chips	92	✓	✓	✓	✓
Lupini Hummus	93	✓	✓	✓	✓
Seed Crackers	94	✓	✓	✓	✓
Nori Energy Sticks	96	✓	✓	✓	✓
Easy Peanut Butter Protein Bars	98	✓	✓		✓
Cucumber Avocado Pinwheels	100	✓	✓	✓	✓
Curry Tofu Salad Bites	102	✓	✓	✓	
Falafel Salad	106	✓	✓	✓	✓
Fattoush Salad	107	✓	✓	✓	✓
Carrot Ginger Soup	108		✓	✓	✓
Spicy Coconut Soup	110		✓	✓	
Creamy Cauliflower Soup	112	✓	✓	✓	✓
Warm Kale Salad	114	✓		✓	✓
Portabella and Summer Squash Salad	115	✓	✓	✓	✓
Green Keto Balance Bowl	116	✓	✓	✓	✓
Taco Salad	118	✓		✓	✓
Greek Salad	120	✓	✓	✓	✓
Garlic Ginger Slaw	121	✓	✓	✓	
Mediterranean Zucchini Salad	122	✓	✓	✓	✓
Lemon Pesto Greens	123	✓	✓	✓	✓
Cucumber Salad	124	✓	✓	✓	✓
Chili Tamari Tofu	126	✓	✓	✓	
Tangy Brussels Sprouts with Mushrooms & Walnuts	128	✓		✓	✓

RECIPES	PAGE	⃠	⃠	⃠	⃠
Crispy Broccoli Bites	129	✓	✓	✓	
Sweet Chili Roasted Radishes	130	✓	✓	✓	
Cabbage Rolls	134	✓		✓	✓
Kelp Noodle Pad Thai	136	✓		✓	
Keto Pot Pie	138	✓		✓	✓
Korean BBQ Tacos	140	✓		✓	
Meal Prep Chili	142	✓		✓	
Smashed Bean Sandwiches	143	✓	✓	✓	✓
Black Bean Burgers	144	✓	✓	✓	
Hemp Seed Nuggets	146	✓	✓	✓	✓
Cauliflower Bake	148	✓	✓	✓	✓
Zucchini Bolognese	149	✓		✓	
Zucchini Alfredo	150	✓	✓	✓	✓
Buffalo Jackfruit Tacos	151			✓	✓
Sparkling Ginger Limeade	154	✓	✓	✓	✓
Blackberry Lemonade	156	✓	✓	✓	✓
Coconut Matcha Latte	158		✓	✓	✓
Keto Pumpkin Spice Latte	159		✓	✓	✓
Golden Chai Protein Smoothie	160	✓	✓	✓	✓
Rise & Shine Smoothie	161	✓	✓	✓	✓
Chocolate Almond Butter Cupcakes	162			✓	✓
Keto Black Bean Brownies	164	✓	✓	✓	
Chocolate Keto Nice Cream	166		✓	✓	✓
Snickerdoodles	168			✓	✓
Sausage Spice Blend	172	✓	✓	✓	✓
Chai Spice Blend	173	✓	✓	✓	✓
Everything Bagel Blend	174	✓	✓	✓	✓
Savory Herb Blend	175	✓	✓	✓	✓
Nut & Seed Flours	176	✓	O	✓	✓
Cauliflower Rice	178	✓	✓	✓	✓
Zucchini Noodles	179	✓	✓	✓	✓
Flax Tortillas	180	✓	✓	✓	✓
Flax Egg	182	✓	✓	✓	✓
Tangy Avocado Mayo	183	✓	✓	✓	✓
Easy Mustard Vinaigrette	184	✓	✓	✓	✓
Quick Hemp Seed Sour Cream	185	✓	✓	✓	✓
Tahini Dressing	186	✓	✓	✓	✓
Keto Buttery Spread	187			✓	✓
Greek Dressing	188	✓	✓	✓	✓
Easy Vegan Pesto	189	✓	✓	✓	✓
Creamy Hemp Sauce	190	✓	✓	✓	✓
Faux Parm Sprinkles	191	✓		✓	✓

General Index